Jenny Markov

Marker-vaccinated animals: A risk of importing the disease or not?

AF063454

Jenny Markov

Marker-vaccinated animals: A risk of importing the disease or not?

Risk assessment concerning the import of marker-vaccinated animals into Switzerland

Südwestdeutscher Verlag für Hochschulschriften

Impressum/Imprint (nur für Deutschland/ only for Germany)
Bibliografische Information der Deutschen Nationalbibliothek: Die Deutsche Nationalbibliothek verzeichnet diese Publikation in der Deutschen Nationalbibliografie; detaillierte bibliografische Daten sind im Internet über http://dnb.d-nb.de abrufbar.
Alle in diesem Buch genannten Marken und Produktnamen unterliegen warenzeichen-, marken- oder patentrechtlichem Schutz bzw. sind Warenzeichen oder eingetragene Warenzeichen der jeweiligen Inhaber. Die Wiedergabe von Marken, Produktnamen, Gebrauchsnamen, Handelsnamen, Warenbezeichnungen u.s.w. in diesem Werk berechtigt auch ohne besondere Kennzeichnung nicht zu der Annahme, dass solche Namen im Sinne der Warenzeichen- und Markenschutzgesetzgebung als frei zu betrachten wären und daher von jedermann benutzt werden dürften.

Verlag: Südwestdeutscher Verlag für Hochschulschriften Aktiengesellschaft & Co. KG
Dudweiler Landstr. 99, 66123 Saarbrücken, Deutschland
Telefon +49 681 37 20 271-1, Telefax +49 681 37 20 271-0, Email: info@svh-verlag.de
Zugl.: Zürich, Veterinärmedizinische Fakultät der Universität Zürich, Inaugural-Dissertation, 2007

Herstellung in Deutschland:
Schaltungsdienst Lange o.H.G., Berlin
Books on Demand GmbH, Norderstedt
Reha GmbH, Saarbrücken
Amazon Distribution GmbH, Leipzig
ISBN: 978-3-8381-0496-6

Imprint (only for USA, GB)
Bibliographic information published by the Deutsche Nationalbibliothek: The Deutsche Nationalbibliothek lists this publication in the Deutsche Nationalbibliografie; detailed bibliographic data are available in the Internet at http://dnb.d-nb.de.
Any brand names and product names mentioned in this book are subject to trademark, brand or patent protection and are trademarks or registered trademarks of their respective holders. The use of brand names, product names, common names, trade names, product descriptions etc. even without a particular marking in this works is in no way to be construed to mean that such names may be regarded as unrestricted in respect of trademark and brand protection legislation and could thus be used by anyone.

Publisher:
Südwestdeutscher Verlag für Hochschulschriften Aktiengesellschaft & Co. KG
Dudweiler Landstr. 99, 66123 Saarbrücken, Germany
Phone +49 681 37 20 271-1, Fax +49 681 37 20 271-0, Email: info@svh-verlag.de

Copyright © 2009 by the author and Südwestdeutscher Verlag für Hochschulschriften Aktiengesellschaft & Co. KG and licensors
All rights reserved. Saarbrücken 2009

Printed in the U.S.A.
Printed in the U.K. by (see last page)
ISBN: 978-3-8381-0496-6

Aus dem
Bundesamt für Veterinärwesen
Direktor: Dr. H. Wyss

und dem

Virologischen Institut der Vetsuisse-Fakultät Universität Zürich
Direktor: Prof. Dr. M. Ackermann

Arbeit unter Leitung von PD Dr. M. Engels und Dr. E. Breidenbach

Risk assessment concerning the import of marker-vaccinated animals into Switzerland

INAUGURAL-DISSERTATION

zur Erlangung der Doktorwürde der
Vetsuisse-Fakultät Universität Zürich

vorgelegt von

Jennifer Zora Markov

Tierärztin
von Winterthur ZH

genehmigt auf Antrag von

Prof. Dr. M. Ackermann, Referent

PD Dr. K. Stärk, Korreferentin

Zürich 2006

To my parents Kathrin and Gawril

Contents

CONTENTS I

LIST OF ABBREVIATIONS V

DEFINITION OF TERMS VII

SUMMARY 1
    Summary in English 1
    Zusammenfassung in Deutsch 1

CHAPTER 1   INTRODUCTION 3

CHAPTER 2   REVIEW OF EXISTING INFORMATION 5
    2.1.   Herpesviruses 5
        2.1.1.   General characteristics 5
            2.1.1.1.   Classification 5
            2.1.1.2.   Replication of alpha-herpesviruses 6
            2.1.1.3.   Pathogenesis of alpha-herpesviruses 6
            2.1.1.4.   Epidemiology of alpha-herpesviruses 7
        2.1.2.   Aujeszky's disease 7
            2.1.2.1.   Agent and disease 7
            2.1.2.2.   Epidemiology 8
        2.1.3.   Infectious bovine rhinotracheitis 8
            2.1.3.1.   Agent and disease 8
            2.1.3.2.   Epidemiology 9
    2.2.   Marker vaccines and DIVA strategies 10
        2.2.1.   DIVA strategies for herpesviruses 12
        2.2.2.   AD marker vaccines 12
        2.2.3.   IBR marker vaccines 12
    2.3.   Eradication programmes for AD and IBR 13
        2.3.1.   AD eradication programmes in Europe 16
        2.3.2.   IBR eradication programmes in Europe 18

- 2.4. International trade standards regarding AD and IBR 19
  - 2.4.1. OIE Standards 19
    - 2.4.1.1. Terrestrial Animal Health Code: Aujeszky's disease 19
    - 2.4.1.2. Terrestrial Animal Health Code: IBR 19
  - 2.4.2. EU standards and Commission decisions 20
    - 2.4.2.1. Trade regulations for Aujeszky's disease 20
    - 2.4.2.2. Trade regulations for IBR 21
  - 2.4.3. Import regulations of Switzerland 23
    - 2.4.3.1. Import regulations for pigs 23
    - 2.4.3.2. Import regulations for cattle 26
- 2.5. Risk analysis for international trade 29

CHAPTER 3 MATERIAL & METHODS 31

- 3.1. Risk assessment 31
- 3.2. Scenario trees 31
- 3.3. Literature research and eliciting expert opinion 32
- 3.4. Model and software 32
- 3.5. Model for Aujeszky's disease 33
  - 3.5.1. Risk profile 33
    - 3.5.1.1. Aim of model and assessment 33
    - 3.5.1.2. Possible hazards 33
    - 3.5.1.3. Endangered values 33
    - 3.5.1.4. Assumptions 33
  - 3.5.2. Scenario tree 34
    - 3.5.2.1. Release assessment Aujeszky's disease 34
    - 3.5.2.2. Exposure assessment Aujeszky's disease 36
  - 3.5.3. Overview and used parameters 38
  - 3.5.4. Input values and calculations 41
    - 3.5.4.1. Node 1: Animal vaccinated 41
    - 3.5.4.2. Node 2: Herd immunity 41
    - 3.5.4.3. Node 3: Animal status 41
    - 3.5.4.4. Node 4: Seroconversion at time of testing 43
    - 3.5.4.5. Node 5: Test abroad 44
    - 3.5.4.6. Node 6: Reactivation at import 45
    - 3.5.4.7. Node 7: Clinical signs 45
    - 3.5.4.8. Node 8: Reactivation lifetime 46
    - 3.5.4.9. Node 9: Transmission of virus 46

3.5.5. Submodels 47
    3.5.5.1. Submodel Herd prevalence (Submodel for node 3).................. 47
    3.5.5.2. Bayes model (Submodel for node 5) 51

3.6. Model for Infectious bovine rhinotracheitis 53

3.6.1. Risk profile 53
    3.6.1.1. Aim of model and assessment.. 53
    3.6.1.2. Possible hazards 53
    3.6.1.3. Endangered values... 53
    3.6.1.4. Assumptions 53

3.6.2. Scenario tree... 54
    3.6.2.1. Release assessment 54
    3.6.2.2. Exposure assessment 56

3.6.3. Overview and used parameters 58

3.6.4. Inputs and calculations for the IBR model....................................... 62
    3.6.4.1. Node 1: Animal vaccinated 62
    3.6.4.2. Node 2: Herd immunity 62
    3.6.4.3. Node 3: Age... 62
    3.6.4.4. Node 4: Animal status... 63
    3.6.4.5. Node 5: Seroconversion.. 67
    3.6.4.6. Node 6: Seroconversion in 21 days.. 67
    3.6.4.7. Node 7: Test abroad 69
    3.6.4.8. Node 8: Separation group size 69
    3.6.4.9. Node 9: Reactivation during import 69
    3.6.4.10. Node 10: Test CH 70
    3.6.4.11. Node 11: Reactivation at introduction....................................... 72
    3.6.4.12. Node 12: Test sentinels 72
    3.6.4.13. Node 13: Reactivation lifetime 73
    3.6.4.14. Node 14: Transmission 74

3.7. Sensitivity analysis 74

CHAPTER 4 RESULTS 75

4.1. Model output.. 75

4.1.1. Aujeszky's disease.. 75

4.1.2. Infectious bovine rhinotracheitis... 77

4.2. Sensitivity analysis 79

4.2.1. Aujeszky's disease.. 79

4.2.2. Infectious bovine rhinotracheitis... 80

CHAPTER 5 DISCUSSION 83

    5.1. Sources of information for the presented models 83

    5.2. Modelling approach 83

        5.2.1. Interpretation of the model outputs 84

        5.2.2. Sensitivity analysis 86

        5.2.3. Different scenarios 88

    5.3. Recommendations for decision-makers 89

REFERENCES 91

INDEX OF TABLES AND FIGURES 101

ACKNOWLEDGEMENTS 103

CURRICULUM VITAE ....FEHLER! TEXTMARKE NICHT DEFINIERT.

List of abbreviations

ACERSA	Association pour la certification de la santé animale (France)
AD	Aujeszky's disease
AHAW	Animal Health and Welfare panel
APP	Actinobacillus pleuropneumoniae
BoHV-1	Bovine herpesvirus type 1
BVD	Bovine virus diarrhea
CSF	Classical swine fever
DIVA	Differentiate infected from vaccinated animals
EC	European Commission
EFSA	European Food Safety Authority
ELISA	Enzyme-linked immunosorbent assay
EP	Swine enzootic pneumonia (mycoplasma hyopneumoniae infection)
EU	European Union
FMD	Foot-and-mouth disease
IBR	Infectious bovine rhinotracheitis
IPV / IPB	Infectious pustular vulvovaginits / infectious pustular balanophostitis
OIE	World Organisation for Animal Health (office international des epizooties)
PCR	Polymerase chain reaction
PRRS	Porcine reproductive and respiratory syndrome
PRV	Pseudorabies virus / suid herpesvirus type 1
R_0	Basic reproductive ratio
SFVO	Swiss Federal Veterinary Office
SPS agreement	Sanitary and phytosanitary measures agreement
SUISAG	Swiss pig breeders organisation
$TCID_{50}$	50% tissue culture infective dose
TRACES	Trade control and expert system
TVD	Swiss national animal movements database (Tierverkehrsdatenbank)
WTO	World Trade Organisation

Definition of terms

Commodity **	Animals, products of animal origin intended for human consumption, for animal feeding, for pharmaceutical or surgical use or for agricultural or industrial use, semen, embryos / ova, biological products and pathological material
Domestic animal	Animal of the domestic herd (i.e. any pig / cattle hold in Switzerland that is not imported)
Domestic herd	Swiss national herd (i.e. all pigs / cattle hold in Switzerland that is not imported)
gB	Glycoprotein B, an envelope protein of herpesviruses
gB-ELISA	Diagnostic kit to detect antibodies against gB in infected cattle (applied to non-vaccinated cattle)
gE	Glycoprotein E, an envelope protein of herpesviruses (suitable to create deletion mutants for marker vaccines)
gE-ELISA	Diagnostic kit to detect antibodies against gE in vaccinated and infected animals (applied to vaccinated animals)
Hazard **	Any pathogenic agent that could produce adverse consequences on the importation or a commodity
Import	Within this thesis, 'import' refers to trade from any country into Switzerland
Indirect ELISA	Conventional diagnostic kit to detect antibodies against BoHV-1 antigens and PRV antigens, respectively (applied to non-vaccinated cattle)
Input *	Any information that is fed into a model (including parameters, variables, data, distributions)
Marker vaccine	Vaccine that allows for DIVA strategy
Model *	A simplified representation of the reality to simulate the biological processes under study
Parameter *	A numerical descriptive measure that characterises a population, mostly used to represent arguments of mathematical, statistical or probability distribution functions
Probability	Likelihood of occurrence of a defined situation
Proportion	Fraction of the population that fulfills defined conditions
PRV-ELISA	Conventional diagnostic kit to detect antibodies against PRV in infected pigs (applied to non-vaccinated pigs)

Risk **	Likelihood of the occurrence and the likely magnitude of the consequences of an adverse event to animal or human health in the importing country, i.e. Switzerland, during a specified time period
Test performance	Sensitivity and specificity of a diagnostic test
Vaccinated	Within this thesis, 'vaccinated' refers to an animal vaccinated with a marker vaccine
Variable *	Any characteristic that has different value for different subjects or objects

* from the OIE handbook (Anonymous, 2004c)
** from the OIE code (Anonymous, 2005e)

Summary

SUMMARY IN ENGLISH

Two risk assessments using stochastic modelling technique were conducted regarding the hypothetical import of marker-vaccinated animals from countries where an official eradication programme was in place. By using scenario trees and collecting information from literature and experts, models were developed for Aujeszky's disease (AD) and Infectious bovine rhinotracheitis (IBR), respectively. The aim of the project was to provide decision makers and risk management with recommendations for possible future import scenarios.

The model for Aujeszky's disease in pigs, using parameters based on an assumed import from the example region Spain, showed for a single imported pig a probability of introduction and subsequent infection of a Swiss pig of 4.9×10^{-4} for a marker-vaccinated and 4.73×10^{-7} for a non-vaccinated pig. For IBR in cattle, using parameters based on an assumed import from Saxony-Anhalt, the model output was for a single imported cattle a probability of introduction and infection of a Swiss cattle of 2.40×10^{-3} for marker-vaccinated and 1.78×10^{-4} for non-vaccinated cattle. Based on these results, import restrictions for vaccinated animals are justified.

The results were strongly dependent from the level of virus presence in the exporting country. Test performance was only relevant in the IBR model since cattle were tested more than once. The probability of seronegative carriers and the probability of reactivation during separation had also an impact on the outcome. For IBR, additional information regarding test dependence and transmission probabilities from vaccinated to non-vaccinated animals would allow for a more precise estimate.

ZUSAMMENFASSUNG IN DEUTSCH

Zwei Risikoabschätzungen bezüglich des hypothetischen Imports von mit Markerimpfstoffen geimpften Tieren aus Ländern mit offiziellem Eradikationsprogramm wurden durchgeführt. Mittels Szenario-Bäumen und Literaturrecherchen sowie Expertenmeinungen wurden zwei stochastische Modelle entwickelt betreffend Aujeszkyscher Krankheit (AD) und Infektiöser boviner Rhinotracheitis (IBR). Das Ziel des Projekts war es, dem Risikomanagement eine Entscheidungshilfe mit Empfehlungen zu zukünftigen Importszenarios zur Verfügung zu stellen.

Das Modell für AD in aus Spanien importierten Schweinen zeigte für ein einzelnes importiertes Schwein eine Wahrscheinlichkeit, die Krankheit einzuschleppen und ein Schweizer Tier zu infizieren von 4.9×10^{-4} für mit Markerimpfstoffen geimpfte und 4.73×10^{-7} für ungeimpfte. Bezüglich IBR in Rindern aus Sachsen-Anhalt waren die Resultate für ein einzelnes importiertes Rind 2.40×10^{-3} für geimpfte und 1.78×10^{-4} für ungeimpfte. Diese Resultate stützen die aktuellen Importbeschränkungen für geimpfte Tiere.

Die Werte waren für beide Modelle stark abhängig von der mengenmässigen Präsenz des Erregers im Exportland. Die Leistungsfähigkeit des Tests war nur für das IBR-Model von Bedeutung, da die Rinder mehrfach getestet werden. Die Wahrscheinlichkeit des Vorkommens seronegativer Träger sowie der Reaktivierung während der Absonderung hatten ebenfalls einen Einfluss. Zusätzliche Informationen zur Abhängigkeit der beiden IBR Tests und zur Übertragungswahrscheinlichkeit zwischen geimpften und ungeimpften Tieren würden eine genauere Schätzung erlauben.

Chapter 1   Introduction

Switzerland is free from a number of infectious diseases in livestock that do still occur in many of the countries from which live animals might be imported. For example, Switzerland is recognized as free from Aujeszky's disease (AD) and infectious bovine rhinotracheitis (IBR) as documented in the annual report of Swiss Federal Veterinary Office (SFVO) (Reist et al., 2006). At the same time, these diseases do occur in at least parts of many European countries, e.g. Germany and France. Some of these countries pursue control programmes targeted at these diseases.

In veterinary medicine, sanitary measures may consist of vaccinating against a certain disease as a method of prevention or eliminating the infection using slaughtering methods such as "stamping out" which is, for many diseases, recommended by the OIE. Major changes in future disease control are nevertheless foreseen, in particular since the devastating outbreak of foot-and-mouth disease (FMD) in the UK in 2001. An important factor is the change in public perception of animal husbandry making slaughtering policies less and less popular. Unfortunately, many veterinary vaccines prevent clinical signs of disease but wild-type virus excretion and spreading of the disease after field infection can still occur (Pastoret, 1999).

In recent years, molecular biology procedures have had a major impact on the preparation of veterinary vaccines, in particular in food animals (Babiuk, 2002; van Oirschot, 1999; van Oirschot et al., 1997). Marker vaccines are newly developed vaccines, which can be used in the scope of a disease elimination program since they allow differentiating between infected from vaccinated animals. "True" marker vaccines are obtained either by the deletion of a certain gene coding for a non-essential protein of the infectious virus (gene deletion vaccines) or by the expression of the major antigenic protein (subunit vaccines) such as the E2 vaccine against classical swine fever (CSF) (van Oirschot, 2001; Moormann et al., 2000).

The crucial feature of marker vaccines is the differentiation of the antibody response. For an effective marker vaccine virus it is critical that the gene product used does not affect its immunogenicity, is expressed in field virus, and is itself a good immunogen. So far, only AD and IBR marker vaccines have been successfully used in the field (van Oirschot, 2001). A CSF marker vaccine has been registered recently in the EU for emergency use, and has been applied in the field in Mexico since 2001 (Depner, K., personal communication). Marker vaccines must always be used together with a companion diagnostic test allowing the distinction between animals infected with the wild-type virus and vaccinated animals. These tests are usually based on the enzyme-linked immunoassay (ELISA) principle.

Until today, Switzerland has not allowed the importation of live animals that are seropositive due to vaccination against a disease exotic to Switzerland even if a marker vaccine was used. However, according to WTO and SPS agreements, international trade may only be restricted if an unacceptable risk to the importing country can be demonstrated using risk assessment methods (Anonymous, 1998). Risk assessments are conducted in the context of international trade according to the guidelines of the OIE (Anonymous, 2004c) and have been successfully used in Switzerland to adapt import requirements (Breidenbach et al., 2004; Hauser et al., 2004).

The objective of the present thesis was to compare the probabilities of introduction of AD and IBR into Switzerland by the import of marker-vaccinated and non-vaccinated live animals, respectively. Therefore, trading regulations and current import practice for pigs and cattle imported from countries not free from the respective infection were examined. The probabilities of introduction were estimated using scenario tree and stochastic modelling techniques, taking into account all available information on biological pathways and test performances. The assessment was conducted to provide decision-makers and risk management with recommendations concerning the possible import of marker-vaccinated animals into Switzerland.

According to the OIE guidelines, risk assessment consists of hazard identification, development of a risk model, including release and exposure assessment as well as consequence assessment. The hazards in this project are the herpes viruses causing AD in pigs and IBR in cattle. A risk model was developed including a scenario tree and a stochastic spreadsheet model. The objective of the risk model was to identify all risk pathways that may lead to the undesired event, i.e., disease introduction into Switzerland, which, in this case, was defined as the infection of one single animal of the domestic herd. The model makes it possible to estimate event probabilities along various branches of the scenario tree and the simulation of various risk management scenarios. Within the scope of a doctoral thesis, models were developed for AD and IBR and estimates were made regarding the probability of introducing the disease by hypothetical import of vaccinated animals. Those estimates were compared to the probability of introduction by import of non-vaccinated animals as practised today, since a zero-risk situation can never be reached. The input values were derived from literature data and expert opinion and can be refined later on in the model if it seems appropriate on the basis of newer findings.

Chapter 2   Review of existing information

2.1. HERPESVIRUSES

2.1.1. General characteristics

Herpesviruses are enveloped double-stranded DNA viruses with a diameter of around 120 to 200 nanometers that infect a wide range of vertebrates and at least one invertebrate (the oyster) though many of them infect only a single species. Their most outstanding characteristic is the capability to establish lifelong latency in infected hosts (Flint et al., 2003).

2.1.1.1. Classification

The Herpesviridae family, comprising more than 120 viruses, is divided into the subfamilies alpha-herpesvirinae, beta-herpesvirinae and gamma-herpesvirinae based on their respective pathogenesis of infection and their genetic properties (Flint et al., 2003). Alpha-herpesvirinae are characterized by rapid replication, causing the lysis of the infected cells. The host range is variable but may be quite broad. Alpha-herpesviruses establish latency mainly in neurons of sensory ganglia but other sites of latency seem to be possible. Beta-herpesvirinae replicate slowly and may induce an enlargement of the infected cells (cytomegaly). They have a restricted host range. Latency is established in lymphoreticular cells and in other organs. Gamma-herpesvirinae are characterized by a narrow host range and a predominant specificity for lymphoblastoid cells, where they replicate and establish latency. In addition, they may be specifically adapted to either B- or T-lymphocytes (Engels and Ackermann, 1996).

Table I provides an overview of the most important species and their hosts.

Table I.   Important members of the family Herpesviridae

	Alpha-herpesvirinae	*Beta-herpesvirinae*	*Gamma-herpesvirinae*
Human	**Herpes simplex virus type 1:** fever blisters **Herpes simplex virus type 2:** genital herpes **Varicella-zoster virus:** zoster, chickenpox	**Human herpesvirus type 5:** cytomegaly **Human herpesvirus type 6:** exanthema subitum	**Epstein-Barr virus:** Burkitt's lymphoma **Human herpesvirus type 8:** Kaposi's sarcoma
Cattle	**Bovine herpesvirus type 1:** infectious bovine rhinotracheitis / infectious pustular vulvovaginitis **Bovine herpesvirus type 2:** bovine herpes mammilitis		**Ovine herpesvirus type 2:** malignant catarrhal fever
Pigs	**Suid herpesvirus type 1:** Aujeszky's disease	**Suid herpesvirus type 2:** cytomegaly (rhinitis)	

Horses	Equine herpesvirus type 1: abortion Equine herpesvirus type 3: coital exanthema Equine herpesvirus type 4: rhinopneumonitis		
Dogs	Canine herpesvirus: death in puppies < 3 weeks		
Cats	Feline herpesvirus: rhinopneumonitis, feline upper respiratory disease complex		
Poultry	Marek's disease virus type 1+2: neurolymphomatosis		

Since the present thesis deals with AD and IBR, which are both caused by alpha-herpesvirinae, it will refer only to this particular subfamily.

2.1.1.2. Replication of alpha-herpesviruses

After infection, virions bind to the cell membrane via envelope glycoproteins gB and gC and enter the host cell mediated by gD, gB, gH, and gI. The released nucleocapsids are transported into the nucleus of the host cell, where replication takes place in three phases. The immediate-early proteins (α-proteins), produced in phase α, activate phase β with the production of early proteins (β-proteins). These proteins control DNA replication and the production of enzymes for DNA synthesis. In phase γ, late proteins (γ-proteins) appear which are primarily virion structural proteins and additional proteins needed for virus assembly and particle egress. After modification and processing of the virus compounds in the endoplasmatic reticulum and the Golgi apparatus, new enveloped virus particles are assembled and released by exocytosis (Flint et al., 2003).

2.1.1.3. Pathogenesis of alpha-herpesviruses

After primary infection, as in many viral diseases, a productive phase with large-scale virus replication leads to acute disease and fast spread of the infection. However, after the host organism has recovered from symptomatic disease, the virus is not eliminated. It remains present in a latent phase.

Latency is characterised by the fact that no infectious virus can be isolated and no viral antigen can be demonstrated in the latently infected cells but viral DNA can be shown by in-situ hybridisation or PCR. Latent infection occurs primarily in neurons found in sensory and autonomic ganglia. Virions enter the host cell as described above but the normal transcription cascade is blocked by yet unknown mechanisms. In the latent state, transcription is severely restricted such that a single pre-mRNA is produced from the latency-associated transcript (LAT) gene. Whether the LATs are translated into proteins remains unclear, but no viral antigens are synthesised. LAT deletion mutants are able to establish latency, but in-vivo experiments indicated that the deletion mutants, in contrast to wild-type virus, showed retarded and less efficient reactivation from latency (Engels and Ackermann, 1996; Rock, 1993).

The interactions between virus, host cell and immune system during latency and reactivation are extremely intricate and still unclear. The mechanism of reactivation of latent infection is not yet thoroughly understood, but the trigger is physical and mental stress (Thiry et al., 1987; Thiry et al., 1985). Furthermore, it is emphasised in the literature that not only the virus but also the host contributes significantly to the efficiency of reactivation (Engels and Ackermann, 1996). However, the stressful situation needed to induce reactivation is simulated in experiments with dexamethasone treatment (Rock et al., 1992; Pastoret et al., 1980; Wellemans et al., 1976).

2.1.1.4. Epidemiology of alpha-herpesviruses

Infection occurs aerogenically, orally or by contact of mucous membranes and virus is excreted mainly via nasal discharge and saliva. Herpesviruses are not very stable in the environment and have low survivability outside of a host. During primary infection, they are disseminated within susceptible populations, spread widely due to an efficient replication mechanism producing high titres of infectious virus but at the same time trigger strong immune responses. In most cases, the population overcomes the disease but retains a long-term reservoir of latent virus carriers. This capability to establish persistent lifelong latency after primary infection that can reactivate and cause new outbreaks of disease is the key to the effectiveness of the viruses double-track strategy (Flint et al., 2003; Engels and Ackermann, 1996)

2.1.2. Aujeszky's disease

2.1.2.1. Agent and disease

The causative agent for AD, suid herpesvirus type 1 (PRV), belongs to the genus varicellovirus within the subfamily alpha-herpesvirinae. Survivability in the environment is comparatively high, even pH-values from 4.0 to 11.0 as reached during curing or decay inactivate the pathogen only slowly (Liess, 1997). The infectious dose for susceptible pigs is reported between 10^2 - 10^4 TCID$_{50}$ (50% tissue culture infective dose), for young piglets only 10^1 TCID$_{50}$ (Visser, 1997) while virus excretion is estimated at 10^6 - 10^9 TCID$_{50}$ in newly infected pigs and around $10^{3.7}$ TCID$_{50}$ in latently infected pigs after reactivation (Wittmann et al., 1982).

AD, also called Pseudorabies or mad itch, was first described by the Hungarian veterinary pathologist Aujeszky in 1902. It is caused by the suid herpesvirus type 1 known as Pseudorabies virus (PRV), an alpha-herpesvirus with a surprisingly wide host range. In its adapted hosts, the pigs, it induces an infection with lympho-haematogenic and neuronal spread and an affinity to central nervous system and respiratory cells. In many other mammals, with the exception of primates and equids, it causes lethal encephalomyelitis. After appearance of central nervous symptoms, fever and typical pruritus at the site of entrance, the animals die within 1-3 days (Liess, 1997). Cattle, goats, sheep, dogs and cats belong to these dead-end hosts and may indicate infection in a nearby pig shelter (Lake et al., 1990), although in very rare cases survival of dead-end host has been reported (Read and Sinclair, 1988).

In pigs, contrary to its colloquial name, PRV infection causes no pruritus. In adult swine the infection is mostly unapparent but abortions and production deficit cause economic losses in farrow and feeder lots. Disease symptoms depend on the age of the pig. In farrowers, acute or peracute encephalomyelitis leads to anankastic movements, ataxia, convulsions and death within one or two days. Morbidity and lethality in runts up to four weeks of age is near 100%. In farrowers up to two months, lethality is around 40-60%. Feeders from three to five months of age develop fever and vomiting, later lack of coordination, tremor and anankastic movements. If no complications such as aspiration pneumonia occur, the disease subsides after 10-15 days but still causes a weight-gain loss and prolonged feeding periods. In adult sows, PRV infection during gravidity can lead to resorption, mumification or abortion, depending on the time of infection. Lethality in adults is as low as 2-5% (Liess, 1997).

2.1.2.2. Epidemiology

Aerogenic virus transmission between farms is possible (Grant et al., 1994), but the most important way of introduction into a herd is the acquisition of latently infected animals. Transmission via contaminated objects like tools, car wheels, or clothing is possible (Weigel et al., 1992). In particular, the use of insufficiently disinfected transport vehicles, journeys to market places or exhibitions with presence of infected pigs and collective transports that visit several farms have been demonstrated as risk factors of disease introduction (Bech-Nielsen et al., 1995; Austin et al., 1993). Other risk factors are pig density in the region, distance to the next pig holding, purchase of gilts, large herd size, and type of holding (Tamba et al., 2002; Leontides et al.,1995; Leontides et al., 1994a; Leontides et al., 1994b; Weigel et al., 1992). Rigorous hygienic measures at the husbandry site and replacement with homebred gilts are negatively associated with disease incidence (Boelaert et al., 1999).

In endemic regions, piglets are protected by maternal antibodies and become susceptible at 6-8 weeks of age when they can survive the disease and subsequently serve as latently infected hosts for the virus. Where the disease is endemic, infection remains mostly unapparent, but takes its toll in the form of production losses due to abortions and stillbirths in breeding animals as well as reduced daily weight gain and secondary respiratory infections in feeder pigs. Furthermore, recurrent losses in other livestock or pet animals associated with pig shelters occur (Salwa, 2004).

In non-endemic regions, the introduction of virus into an uninfected establishment can be devastating. Outbreaks in breeding farms can lead to nearly complete loss of a whole production cycle due to gravidity disorders, stillbirth and lethal disease in farrowers. In feeder farms, there are fewer deaths, but weight losses prolong feeding periods and generate additional costs. And obviously, treatment costs and disinfection of holdings increase the economic impact.

As in many pig diseases, wild boars must be considered as a potential hazard especially in regions where outdoor raising allows contacts between domestic pigs and wild boars. In Germany, seroprevalence of AD in wild boars reaches 25% and higher in endemic areas (Muller et al., 1998b) and a survey during two regular hunting seasons in 2004 -2005 in Switzerland showed prevalences ranging from 0 to 3.73% in 1060 sampled wild boars (Koeppel et al., 2006). On the other hand, recent research has shown differences between circulating virus strains. Viruses isolated from wild boars have shown only low virulence in domestic pigs and vice versa (Muller et al., 2000; Muller et al., 1998a). Furthermore, measures are taken to prevent contacts between outdoor raising pigs and wild boars and during a survey in 2004 there was no evidence of AD found in outdoor pigs (Koeppel et al., 2006). This way of transmission route is therefore thought negligible although possible and not further considered in the present thesis.

2.1.3. Infectious bovine rhinotracheitis

2.1.3.1. Agent and disease

The infectious agent, Bovine herpesvirus type 1 (BoHV-1), is a member of the subfamily of alpha-herpesvirinae, genus varicellovirus. It codes for at least 10 envelope glycoproteins (van Drunen Littel-van den Hurk et al., 2001) which are important targets for the host immune response (Anonymous, 2005b). Although lower than PRV, survivability in the environment is comparatively high. In a cold and humid environment, virions may remain infectious for about one month and resist pH-values from 6.0 to 9.0. After infection of non-vaccinated cattle, excretion of virus titres up to 10^7 $TCID_{50}$ have been recorded and after reactivation of latent infection titres of $10^{1.5}$ $TCID_{50}$ are still reached which can be enough to infect another non-vaccinated herd mate (Hage et al., 1996). Thus, the minimal infective dose has been estimated at $10^{3.2}$ TCID$_{50}$ in naive cattle (Straub, 1979) and 10^3 TCID$_{50}$ in maternally immune calves (Schynts et al., 2001). Virus excretion is usually limited to the first two weeks of infection (Konig et al., 2003; Straub, 2001).

Different virus strains were isolated and three subtypes (1.1, 1.2a and 1.2b) have been identified (Smith et al., 1995; Engels et al., 1986). Nevertheless, all strains are serologically identical and can only be differentiated by means of restriction endonuclease profiles.

BoHV-1 infection is widespread in cattle all over the world. It has first been described in 1950 in the United States and later caused actual epidemics in the 1960s and 70s in European countries. The first outbreak in Switzerland was recorded in 1978/79 (Ackermann et al., 1989). BoHV-1 causes a range of diseases in cattle, including classical IBR and abortion, which are of greatest economic impact, and IPV/IPB (Anonymous, 2005b; Straub, 1990). The clinical signs range from sub-clinical infection to mild or severe disease, depending on virus strain, immunological status of the host, age of the animal, and environmental factors (Pritchard et al., 2003). Other possible symptoms are metritis, mastitis and dermatitis as well as lethal meningoencephalitis and enteritis in young calves.

IBR, the respiratory form of BoHV-1 infection, manifests itself as an acute febrile disease accompanied by nasal discharge and conjunctivitis (van Drunen Littel-van den Hurk et al., 2001). As with other herpesvirus infections, mortality is much higher in young animals. It causes weight-losses and may lead to death, especially among young calves and newborn animals. Particularly in feedlots with cattle less than one year of age, it is associated with the bovine respiratory disease complex, also referred to as shipping fever, which is caused by several bovine viruses and secondary bacterial infections (van Drunen Littel-van den Hurk, 2006). Due to its ability to modify the upper respiratory tract tissues and to cause immunomodulation, BoHV-1 is considered to be one of the major initiators of the disease (Makoschey and Keil, 2000). In adults, infection with BoHV-1 causes high fever, conjunctivitis, nasal discharge, sudden reduction of milk production, but only sporadic deaths (van Drunen Littel-van den Hurk, 2006). Abortions and reduced fertility as a result of infection further aggravate the economic losses furthermore (Hage et al., 1996).

In regions where IBR is endemic, sub-clinical infections without visible clinical signs are most common. Calves are protected by maternal antibodies and clinical signs would appear, if ever, only in younger cattle after farrowing. Nevertheless, losses due to abortions, fertility disorders, reduced milk production in dairy cows and reduced weight gain in calves still occur.

2.1.3.2. Epidemiology

Transmission of BoHV-1 usually occurs by direct contact of a susceptible animal with an infected virus-excreting animal. Aerosol spread does occur but is considered to be limited to a few meters in most cases (Mars et al., 2000). Additional transmission routes are via infected semen (Kupferschmied et al., 1986) and vertical transmission (Ludwig, 1983).

New introduction of BoHV-1 into a population leads to fast spread among susceptible hosts, and febrile respiratory tract diseases cause losses in all sectors of cattle production (Vonk Noordegraaf et al., 2000). Due to breeding synchronisation, it may also cause abortion storms, and it has been associated with central nervous disorders as well as with death in newborn calves. Despite the strong immune response, the virus establishes life-long latency in infected hosts and may be reactivated at intervals to cause new outbreaks of disease (Engels and Ackermann, 1996).

Where IBR is endemic, virus spread is mostly unapparent and asymptomatic but economic losses are inevitable. Sporadic outbreaks of abortions and production losses and the association with the bovine respiratory disease complex keep BoHV-1 infections on the list of economically significant diseases in endemic regions as well. Furthermore, there is evidence that field virus infection or vaccination with a live mutant vaccine in calves with high levels of maternal antibody may produce a delay or even absence of active seroconversion (Lemaire et al., 2000a; Lemaire et al., 2000b). For surveillance and eradication programmes, such seronegative carriers might represent a problem.

Up to now, Bovinae, including zebus and buffalos, seem to be the natural hosts of BoHV-1. But infection of sheep, goats, deer (Wyler et al., 1989) and Camelidae (Puntel et al., 1999) may occur and results in mild or unapparent clinical signs. Although, in theory, transmission from acutely infected sheep to cattle could occur upon contact, there is no evidence that any of the non-bovine hosts could act as a long-lasting reservoir (Mollema et al., 2005; Hage et al., 1997).

Acquisition of latently infected animals is the main cause for the introduction of BoHV-1 into a formerly negative herd (van Schaik et al., 2001). Herd size and type of holding are further risk factors for seropositivity and, following, cattle density in the region and distance to closest cattle holding (Magana-Urbina et al., 2005; Dispas et al., 2003). Aerogenic transmission has been reported, but only over short distances (Mars et al., 2000), and contaminated tools, including vaccination syringes, may cause infections. As for AD, contaminated and insufficiently disinfected transport vehicles, other contaminated objects, and journeys to exhibitions with presence of infected animals represent risk factors for virus transmission (Boelaert et al., 2005; van Schaik et al., 2001).

2.2. MARKER VACCINES AND DIVA STRATEGIES

Many efforts have been made to combat herpesvirus infections in animals, and vaccination is a common tool in many species. For example, most owners have their cats vaccinated against feline rhinotracheitis (Cocker et al., 1984), and for horses, most breeding associations recommend to vaccinate breeding animals by most breeding associations. In livestock production, vaccination against AD in pigs and IBR in cattle is practiced in many countries worldwide. But it turned out that vaccinated animals, even with strong antibody response, are not protected against infection and latency (Schoenbaum et al., 1990; de Leeuw and van Oirschot, 1985). Clinical protection can be achieved and losses reduced but the virus is still present in the population. Under these conditions a major drawback is the unknown status of an animal after vaccination and vaccination has to be continued to prevent new outbreaks of disease.

To overcome this problem, a method to distinguish between vaccinated and infected animals is very desirable, not only for herpesviruses but also for several other viral infections of importance in livestock production. Such a method can make vaccination a much more valuable tool in eradication programmes despite its deficiency in preventing infection. Thus, a combination of vaccination and removal of infected animals is possible, resulting in a more economical way of expanded eradication (Wittmann, 1991). It has been suggested that marker vaccines need not prevent infection in order to be effective in an eradication programme because reduced susceptibility and reduced transmission can have a major impact on disease prevalence (Henderson, 2005; van Oirschot, 1999). But in emergency situations such as outbreaks of FMD or CSF, marker vaccines could also be of great value. Emergency ring vaccination could be performed without complicating the epidemiological situation, and the spreading of field virus would still be under control. As additional benefit in view of the rising concern among the public, uninfected vaccinated animals would not be subject to culling after emergency vaccination.

Different strategies concerning different infections and virus types have been developed to achieve this aim, but the basic approach is the same. All DIVA-strategies ("differentiate infected from vaccinated animals") include a marker vaccine and a companion diagnostic test. The technique may be as basic as identifying naturally occurring strains with deletions that support differentiating infected from vaccinated animals, but more sophisticated technologies may also be employed. Regardless of the specific method, the diagnostic kit must be able to detect wild-type virus specific immune responses (Henderson, 2005).

Recombinant technologies allow the construction of live virus vectors, such as various pox and adenovirus strains, that express immunogenic proteins from, for example, rabies virus (Roscoe et al., 1998), FMD virus (Moraes et al., 2003), CSF virus (Hahn et al., 2003), West Nile virus (Siger et al., 2004), and avian influenza virus (Swayne et al., 2000). For rabies in foxes, racoons, and coyotes, a positive marker strategy has been used to mark and detect vaccinated animals. This is because in wildlife, monitoring of exposure to vaccine virus is a highly desirable way of assessing the effectiveness of applied measures (Roscoe et al., 1998). By contrast, in livestock where the vaccination status of the animals is usually known, exposure to wild-type virus is of greatest interest. For this reason, negative marker strategies are applied, i.e. infected animals are "marked" and can therefore be detected with the corresponding diagnostic test while vaccinated animals result as "unmarked" negatives in the same test. For example, for CSF, a subunit vaccine containing core protein E2 is combined with an E^{RNS}-blocking ELISA to detect antibodies against non-E2 proteins (Beer and Mettenleiter, 2004; Bouma et al., 2000) as shown in Figure 1. Gene deletions in viruses, whether spontaneous or engineered, can also be used for DIVA-strategies, provided the deletion-mutants can produce sufficient immunity to protect against disease while the deleted gene provokes a reliable additional immune response after infection. Such strategies have been investigated for PRV (Mettenleiter, 2000; van Oirschot et al., 1996b), BoHV-1 (van Oirschot et al., 1996b), and CSF virus strains (Meyers et al., 1999).

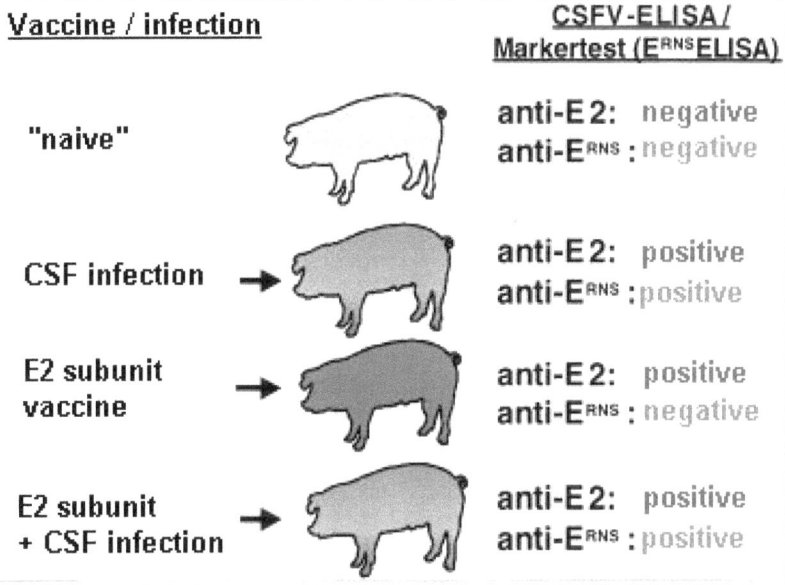

Figure 1. Principles of a CSF subunit marker vaccine
(With kind permission from Beer and Mettenleiter (2004))

The figure shows expected test results for different situations. Naïve animals are negative in any applied test and infected animals are positive in both tests. Marker- vaccinated pigs react positively in the anti-E2-ELISA as they possess antibodies against E2 after E2 subunit vaccination, while they remain negative in the anti-E^{RNS}-ELISA. Only vaccinated animals latently infected with CSF show positive results in the anti-E^{RNS}-ELISA.

2.2.1. DIVA strategies for herpesviruses

For herpesviruses, deletion mutants for several glycoproteins have been developed and tested under experimental conditions (Pensaert et al., 1990). The difficulty was to trigger a sufficient immune response to prevent clinical symptoms and reduce virus transmission and, at the same time keeping the deleted glycoprotein sufficiently immunogenic to assure additional antibody production after wild-type infection. The envelope glycoprotein E (gE), proved to be the ideal candidate (Schwyzer and Ackermann, 1996; van Engelenburg et al., 1994). gE-deletion mutants are able to infect cells and replicate. They trigger a strong immune response but their virulence is minimal and there is minimal virus spread. In wild-type virus, gE is strongly conserved and there where no gE-deletion mutants found in the field. Furthermore, gE provokes an antibody response within reasonable time and the gE-antibodies can be detected in wild-type virus infected animals with ELISA techniques (Beer and Mettenleiter, 2004).

2.2.2. AD marker vaccines

The first licensed genetically engineered vaccine, an AD vaccine (Zuckermann, 2000), was introduced in 1988 with a companion gE-blocking ELISA kit to detect wild-type virus infection (Mellencamp et al., 1989; van Oirschot, 1988a). Several vaccines against AD were already in practice at that time (de Leeuw and van Oirschot, 1985; Vannier, 1985) to minimise economic losses, and the commercially used vaccine strains Bartha, Begonia, and Phylaxia turned out to be gE-deletion mutants anyway (van Oirschot et al., 1990a; van Oirschot et al., 1988c). This circumstance entailed rapid advances in DIVA strategies for AD because purity, potency, safety, and efficacy of those vaccines had already been investigated, and only the performance of the gE-blocking ELISA kits had to be evaluated (Eloit et al., 1989). It was found experimentally that gE-deletion mutants could still cause severe disease or death in three-day-old piglets. To further reduce virulence and decrease the likelihood of reversion to it, mutants with an additional deletion in the thymidine kinase gene were constructed as, for example, the genetically engineered strain 783 (van Oirschot et al., 1991; Moormann et al., 1990; van Oirschot et al., 1990b; Kit et al., 1987). PRV-marker vaccines and companion diagnostic kits have been successfully implemented in many eradication campaigns ever since (Stegeman, 1995; MacDiarmid, 1990) and have been shown to be effective in reducing clinical symptoms after infection, wild-type virus replication after infection, and transmission of wild-type virus in experimental infections and in the field (van Oirschot et al., 1996b; Mettenleiter, 1995)

2.2.3. IBR marker vaccines

Conventional IBR vaccines have been, and still are, routinely used but in many EU member states, their use is prohibited in favour of marker vaccines. Figure 2 shows the principle of such a DIVA strategy. For IBR-marker vaccines like for AD vaccines, gE-deletion mutants are used. One reason is that gE is not essential for replication of the virus in cell cultures. Additionally, no bovine serum is needed to grow them, which reduces the risk of contamination with other bovine viruses. In vivo, gE is an important virulence factor and, in contrast to AD vaccine strains, the deletion of gE is already sufficient to attenuate BoHV-1. So far, no gE-negative virus strains have been isolated from cattle and gE is immunogenic enough to provoke a clear antibody response. As additional advantage, marker vaccines, as opposed to conventional IBR vaccines, are much less likely to be transmitted to non-vaccinated contact animals. The deletion mutants are derived from conventionally attenuated BoHV-1 strains or from genetically engineered viruses (Beer and Mettenleiter, 2004; Makoschey and Lütticken, 2002).

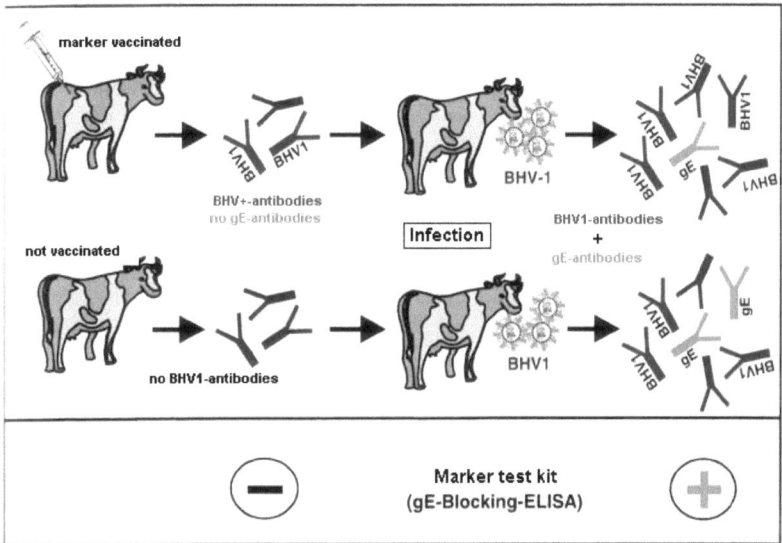

Figure 2. DIVA strategy for IBR (With kind permission from Beer and Mettenleiter (2004))

Marker-vaccinated animals produce BoHV1-antibodies but no gE-antibodies, while non-vaccinated animals have no antibodies against BHV1 at all. In a conventional indirect ELISA and in the modern gB-ELISA, the vaccinated cow would therefore be positive while the non-vaccinated one would remain negative. In the gE-blocking ELISA both animals give a negative result. After infection with wild-type BoHV1, the non-vaccinated animal seroconverts to BoHV1 with a complete antibody spectrum while the vaccinated animal produces gE-antibodies in addition to its BoHV1-antibodies. Now both animals are positive in any applied test and the vaccinated cow can be identified as latently infected using the gE-blocking ELISA.

2.3. ERADICATION PROGRAMMES FOR AD AND IBR

Several devastating animal diseases could be effectively eradicated from livestock populations to protect the human population from important zoonoses or to avoid economic losses in animal production. Bovine tuberculosis, brucellosis, CSF, African swine fever, and FMD are only some examples of successful eradication campaigns in many European countries. In most cases, the strategy includes screening tests and stamping out of infected animals or herds followed by surveillance programmes to maintain disease-free status. For widespread infections, vaccination strategies are also common in the early stage of eradication. After successful eradication, rigorous legal regulations and stringent measures to deal with occasional outbreaks, for example after import of infected animals, as well as positive results in monitoring programmes prevent further spread if the disease should reappear.

Eradication campaigns are expensive and require a functional veterinary service for monitoring and surveillance. Culling or vaccination in large populations requires personnel resources and education, and fair compensation of affected farmers is important. Otherwise, compliance will decrease and all official efforts would be wasted, as freedom from disease cannot be achieved.

In the EU, eradication programmes may be approved by the Commission. For approved programmes, annual financial support from the Community is granted. Table II summarises the situation regarding AD and IBR in Europe in 2004, taking into account information from EU as well as from OIE.

Table II. Situation in the EU member states regarding AD and IBR in 2004

Country	Aujeszky's disease				Infectious bovine rhinotracheitis			
	EU Status [1]	Vaccination	Eradication programme [2]	OIE 2004: [3] Last reported outbreak	EU Status [1]	Vaccination	Eradication programme [2]	OIE 2004: [3] Last reported outbreak
Austria	Free	∅	-	1996	Free	∅	-	2004 19 cases
Belgium	+	✓	02-05	2002	+	x	-	no data
Cyprus	Free	∅	-	1967	+	x	-	no data
Czech Republic	Free	∅	-	2004 1 outbreak (4)	+	✓	-	2004 1 outbr. (295)
Denmark	Free	∅	-	1991	Free	∅	-	2003
Estonia	+	x	-	never		✓	-	2004 serol. evidence
Finland	Free	∅	-	never	Free	∅	-	1994
France	+ (free)	✓	02-05	2004 2 outbreaks	+	✓	-	no data
Germany	Free	x	-	2000	+	✓	04-05	2004 69 outbreaks
Greece	+	x	-	2001	+	x	-	2003
Hungary	+	✓	04-05	2004 serol. evidence	+	✓	-	no data
Ireland	+	✓	03-05	no data	+	x	-	no data
Italy	+	✓	only in Bolzano	2004 1 outbreak (17)	+ (free zone)	✓	-	2002
Latvia	+	✓	-	2004 2 outbreaks (197)	+	✓	-	2004 1 outbreak (20)
Lithuania	+	x	04	1988	+	✓	-	2004 serol. evidence
Luxembourg	Free	∅	-	1999	+	✓	-	2004 serol. evidence
Malta	+	x	04	never	+	x	-	no data
Netherlands	+	✓	02	2004 serol. evidence	+	✓	-	no data
Poland	+	✓	-	2004 21 outbreaks (571)	+	x	-	2004 serol. evidence
Portugal	+	✓	02-05	2004 563 cases (693 cases in wb)	+	✓	-	2004 210 cases

Country								
Slovakia	+	✓	04-05	2004 1outbreak (1952)	+	✓	-	2004 6 outbr. (9963)
Slovenia	+	X	-	2004 serol. evidence	+	✓	-	no data
Spain	+	✓	97-05	2004 2899 (47696)	+	✓	-	2004 1234 (9209)
Sweden	Free	Ø	-	1995	Free	Ø	-	1995
U.K.	Free	Ø	-	1989	+	X	-	2004: 1 case on Isle of Man
(Northern Ireland)	+	✓	-	2004 1 case	+	✓	-	2004 13 outbreaks
Switzerland*	Free	Ø	-	1993	Free	Ø	-	2004 1 outbreak (2)

1		Status according to 2004/EC/320 (AD) and 2004/EC/215 (IBR)
2		Eradication programme approved by EU Commission for the listed years
3		As reported to OIE and published in Handistatus II
*		Not an EU member state but included for completeness of information
+		Country designated as not free, no additional guarantees in intra-community trade
Ø		Vaccination prohibited
✓		Vaccination practiced
X		Not known if vaccination is practiced (not mentioned in OIE Handistatus II)
-		No approved eradication programme implemented
case		Diseased animal
outbreak		Infected establishment with diseased animals
()		Number in brackets represents number of cases reported
wb		Wild boars
serol.		Serological evidence for presence of virus in survey but no cases reported

Switzerland is recognised as free from AD as well as IBR. This is prooven by an annual risk-based survey (Hadorn et. al., 2002b). In the last century, AD has been present in Switzerland (Ehrensperger et. al., 1984) and since 1987, serological investigations were conducted on irregular intervals (Ackermann and Engels, 2003). In 1993, the last positive reactor was identified (Handistatus II, OIE) and in the Agricultural Agreement of 21 June 1999, Switzerland was recognised as free from AD by the EU. To maintain its status, an annual survey providing a 99% confidence that herd level prevalence is below 0.1% is required. Therefore, since 2001, surveys are conducted regularly (Hadorn et. al., 2002a) and no reactors were found up to now. Under the bilateral agreement with the EU, Switzerland can request additional guarantees concerning AD for imported live pigs.

Concerning IBR, the last important outbreak in Switzerland was in 1978/79 whithin the spread of BoHV-1 over whole Europe in the 60s and 70s (Ackermann et. al., 1989; Ackermann et. al., 1990a). Due to rigouros sanitation measures (Ackermann et. al., 1990b), Switzerland could eradicate IBR and became recognised as free by the EU in the Agricultural agreement of 21 June 1999. Nevertheless, sporadic cases still occur due to contact to infected animals abroad (border grazing areas, exhibitions etc.) or artificial insemination with infected semen (Kupferschmied et. al., 1986; Hofmann-Lehmann et. al., 2004). To maintain the disease free status of Switzerland, all cases are thoroughly investigated and the establishment is put under movement ban until all positive reactors are culled. Additionally, an annual survey providing 99% confidence that herd level prevalence is below 0.1% is requested by the EU. Within these surveys, establishments that harbour imported animals are targeted (Reist et. al., 2006). As a consequence of its status, Switzerland can request additional guarantees concerning IBR for imported live cattle.

2.3.1. AD eradication programmes in Europe

Due to the devastating effects in young pig populations and in dead-end hosts such as cattle, eradication of AD is a highly desirable goal and has been started in many European countries within the last 25 years. By now, nine EU member countries, as well as Switzerland and Norway, have achieved freedom from disease while eleven states are in the process of eradication (Figure 3). Although other efforts on the part of breeding associations or producer organisations may exist to fight the disease in the remaining countries, only official eradication programmes approved by the EC are considered in the present thesis. For these official programmes, all details on strategy and current disease situation are provided as reports to the EU, whereas reliable data on other programmes might not be readily available. Table III describes some of the approved programmes in EU member states.

Many strategies are applied in the approved eradication programmes, depending on prevalences, economic impact and available resources. In Malta, where the disease has never been reported, a monitoring programme is implemented to demonstrate freedom from disease. Only one country, Lithuania, follows a strict detection and culling strategy, while in the other nine programmes, eradication is supported by marker vaccination to avoid mass culling and large economic losses. Still, detection and stamping out of seemingly healthy virus carriers is inevitable in the eradication of herpesviruses but difficult to communicate to stakeholders. In this situation, marker vaccination to diminish virus circulation and stepwise culling of reactors can be very helpful although vaccinated animals may still become infected.

In the nine countries with vaccination strategies, vaccines other than marker vaccines are prohibited. Where vaccination is compulsory, breeding pigs must be vaccinated three times per year while for fatteners either one or two vaccinations are administered. Corresponding to the high vaccination frequency and the fast production cycles, screening tests are conducted up to three times per year with gE-ELISAs and negative herds are officially certified as free from disease. Normally, only a subset of animals in a herd is tested to prove the negative status of the herd at a certain confidence level and threshold. Positive results are retested with confirmatory tests to avoid needless culling. In some programmes, vaccination may be terminated in individual hers when they are free from disease. In this case, certification of disease-free herds includes two stages, free with and without vaccination.

The problem in eradication strategies involving vaccination is when to terminate vaccination. For freedom from disease status in international trade, vaccination has to be prohibited. But terminating vaccination too early can render all efforts useless if virus circulation starts again. Some countries, although free from gE-positive reactors for years, are unwilling to stop compulsory vaccination as long as virus is still present in the neighbouring countries. Especially for these countries, export restrictions represent a major burden and might not be needed.

Table III. Details on some approved AD eradication programmes in Europe in 2004

	Vaccine	Scheme	Test
Belgium	gE-negative only	Breeding pigs: 2x before first service, from the age of 10-14 weeks on Purchased pigs: 2x within 4 weeks Gilts: 3x per year (mlv)/ 2x per year (inact.) Fatteners: min. 1x	HerdCheck (gE-ELISA)
Hungary	gE-negative only		gE-ELISA
Ireland	gE-negative: Porcilis Begonia, Geskypur, Suvaxyn Aujeszky	Weaners: twice Replacement and breeding pigs: 3x Purchased Pigs: Vaccination at entry	gE-ELISA
Portugal	gE-negative only	Fattening pigs: 1x (at 10-12 weeks) Breeding pigs: 3x per year	ELISA
Slovakia	gE-negative: Porcilis Begonia only	only emergency vaccination by official veterinarians, direct slaughter afterwards	gE-ELISA
Spain	gE-negative only	breeding pigs: 3x per year Feeders and breeders: mind. 2x, first vacc. at 10 to 12 weeks	gE-ELISA gB-ELISA

Table III includes only programmes, where more specified information was available. For basic information see Table II.

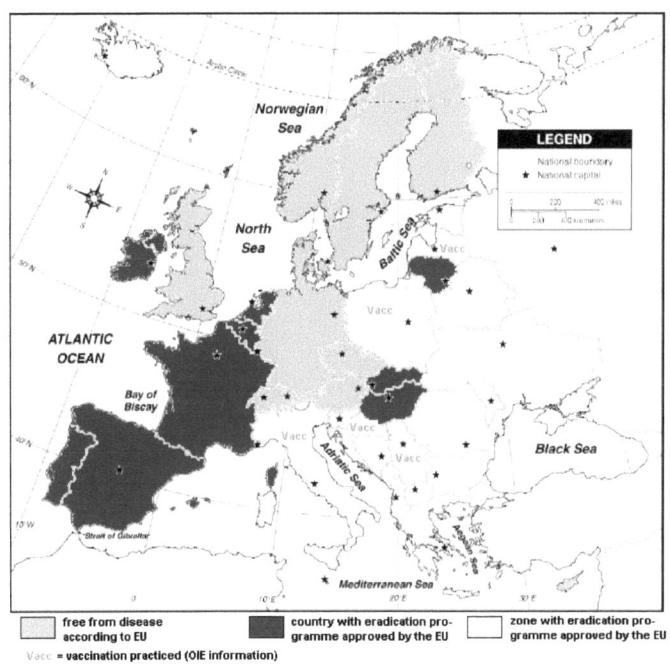

Figure 3. Situation for Aujeszky's disease in Europe 2004 according to 2004/EC/320

2.3.2. IBR eradication programmes in Europe

Europe has a long history of combating against BoHV-1 infection, yet, only a small number of countries have achieved IBR eradication as shown in Figure 4. Currently, these are Switzerland, Norway, Austria, Sweden, Denmark, Finland and the region of Bolzano in Italy. Due to low prevalence at the start of eradication in these countries, a direct test-and-slaughter policy was successfully implemented. In many other countries, measures to eradicate BoHV-1 infection are taken on the part of breeding or trading associations and also at private farm level (Ackermann and Engels, 2006; Anonymous, 2005b). But so far, only one country, Germany, has submitted an official nationwide eradication programme to the EC and obtained additional guarantees in case of import of live cattle from countries not free from IBR. The programme permits marker vaccination but it's not compulsory, and different strategies are applied in the different regions depending on available resources and seroprevalences. Where vaccination is practiced, breeding animals are vaccinated twice a year while fatteners may be vaccinated less frequently. The programme is based on annual testing of all animals to detect and cull seropositive animals. Certification of establishments as free from disease with or without vaccination is possible (Anonymous, 2004b).

For IBR, another strategy, applied in France by ACERSA (Association pour la Certification de la Santé Animale) also merits consideration. In this strategy, vaccination of reactors is permitted. An establishment may be certified as uninfected without or with vaccination (appellation A and B) but vaccination is voluntary for all herds. It is only compulsory if positive reactors older than 24 months are detected but not culled. Those reactors must be vaccinated afterwards (Anonymous, 2005c). Voluntary vaccination leads to herds with variable serostatus and herds where only part of the animals are vaccinated, which represents a situation never investigated under experimental conditions. However, this strategy has so far not been supported by the EU (Anonymous, 2005c).

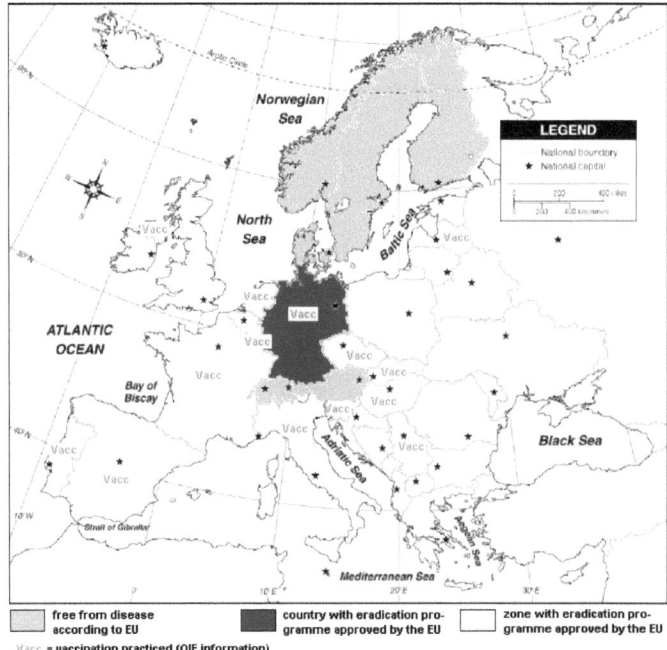

Figure 4. Situation for IBR in Europe 2004 according to 2004/EC/215

2.4. INTERNATIONAL TRADE STANDARDS REGARDING AD AND IBR

International trading of animals and commodities of animal origin is subject to the general WTO guidelines for international trade and, additionally, to the SPS agreement. It is stated that import restrictions may only be imposed if it is demonstrated by the means of risk assessment that the risk for the importing country is greater than in domestic trade. In animals, the possible risks are manifold due to the great number of diseases and zoonoses, and import restrictions may be imposed under international guidelines without conducting a complete risk analysis. OIE recommendations and European law may be considered as guidelines for animal and commodity trade.

2.4.1. OIE Standards

The health standards published by the OIE provide guidelines for trade concerning specific animal diseases. For terrestrial animals, they are contained in the Terrestrial Animal Health Code, Part II, which covers the 'priority' diseases for international trade (OIE list). The aim is to assure the sanitary safety of international trade by detailing health measures to be implemented by the veterinary authorities of importing and exporting countries in order to avoid the transfer of agents pathogenic for animals or humans while avoiding unjustified sanitary barriers. The measures have been formally adopted by the OIE International Commitee, the general assembly of all delegates of OIE member countries, and represent the result of the ongoing work by internationally renowned specialists since 1960. Additionally, OIE provides a manual of diagnostic tests and vaccines for terrestrial animals.

2.4.1.1. Terrestrial Animal Health Code: Aujeszky's disease

In Chapter 2.2.2. of the Terrestrial Animal Health Code definitions and recommendations for AD are given which can be summarised as follows. To export animals from a country or region with a certain status, an international veterinary certificate is required to certify that the pigs fulfil the required conditions. It is always permitted to transfer pigs from an establishment, zone or country with higher status to a destination establishment, zone or country with lower status. On the other hand, for shipment from an infected country to a country with higher status it is recommended to impose a quarantine of 30 days including serological testing and a certificate confirming that the pigs were free from clinical signs of AD, are non-vaccinated, and had been kept in an AD free establishment since birth. For the trade of semen and embryos/ova there exist analogous requirements not specified in this abstract. This chapter of the code is currently under revision.

2.4.1.2. Terrestrial Animal Health Code: Infectious bovine rhinotracheitis

Definitions and recommendations for IBR / IPV are provided in Chapter 2.3.5.1. of the Terrestrial Animal Health Code and can be summarised as follows. To export animals from a country or region with a certain status, an international veterinary certificate is required to certify that the cattle fulfil the required conditions. It is always permitted to transfer cattle from an establishment, zone or country with higher status to a destination establishment, zone or country with lower status. It is recommended to demand a quarantine of 30 days and serological tests on two occasions with an interval of at least 21 days for the transfer of cattle from an infected country to a country with higher health status. Cattle moved from an establishment not free from IBR to another establishment not officially certified as free should be vaccinated according to OIE. For the trade of semen and embryos/ova there exist analogous requirements not specified in this abstract.

2.4.2. EU standards and Commission decisions

While the OIE code makes only recommendations to its member countries, EU Commission decisions are binding for all EU member states, and Switzerland is also subject to the veterinary trade standards under the Bilateral Agreements. For European trade of livestock, "Council Directive 64/432/EEC of 26 June 1964 on animal health problems affecting intra-community trade in bovine animals and swine" and its additional specifications apply. The Council Directive has frequently been amended since 1964, but the document constitutes the basis of all Commission decisions on trade in bovine and swine. The most important update occurred in 1997 with Council Directive 97/12/EC when all additions and amendments for 64/432/EEC were laid down in a new Directive.

The original directive was primarily concerned with zoonoses that threaten human health and for these, compulsory Europe-wide eradication campaigns were implemented. Over the years, more and more diseases of economic impact have been added on a voluntary basis. Annex E, Part I, lists the notifiable diseases that must be monitored in all member states. The respective disease situations, e.g. for bovine tuberculosis and CSF, must be reported annually to the Commission annually (Art.8). For diseases in Annex E, Part II, including AD and IBR, eradication programmes may be approved (Art.9) by the Commission and additional guarantees requested by zones or countries free from disease (Art.10) but all measures are voluntary. Nonetheless, the additional guarantees demanded for international trade may not be stricter than those applied to animal movements within the country itself.

2.4.2.1. Trade regulations for Aujeszky's disease

Already in 1982 the Commission submitted a proposal to the Council to establish trading regulations for AD but no agreement was reached. When 10 years later the situation had become urgent due to the liberalisation of trade in pigs after cessation of vaccination against CSF, an agreement on measures was reached and specific rules were established by Commission Decision 93/24/EEC for pigs entering areas recognised as free from AD. This decision was followed by others concerning approved eradication programmes. Decision 93/244/ECC sets out additional guarantees for pigs entering parts of the Community where an approved eradication programme is in operation and was amended to include other parts where eradication programmes have since been approved.

These decisions have effectively divided the Community into three regions: free areas, areas where approved eradication campaigns are in operation and the remainder where the disease is either not under official control or where eradication programmes are not sufficiently advanced to be approved. On the basis of the Bilateral Agreements, Switzerland is recognised as free from AD and additional guarantees concerning the import of live pigs may be requested from exporting countries.

The conditions for trade were subdivided according to the purpose of the traded pigs: animals for breeding, animals for production and animals for immediate slaughter. In the context of the present thesis, only the conditions regarding breeding pigs will be examined, because only pigs destined to spend the rest of their lifetime in Switzerland pose a possible threat to national population if they are latently infected. In any case, the transfer of pigs to areas of equal health status is possible without restrictions.

Transfer to free areas
- The disease must be notifiable in the country of origin
- No evidence of the disease in the herd of origin during the past 12 months
- The pig must have been held in that establishment since birth
  OR at least during the last 3 months and in others of equivalent status since birth
- Not vaccinated and only gE-deleted vaccines used in the herd of origin within the past 12 months
- Isolated for at least 30 days and tested after 21 days, where all pigs in isolation must be negative in the test

Transfer to areas where an approved eradication programme is in operation
- The disease must be notifiable in the country of origin
- No evidence of the disease in the herd of origin in the past 12 months
- The pig must have been held in that establishment since birth
  OR at least during the last 3 months and in others of equivalent status since birth
- The pig may be vaccinated with a gE-negative vaccine, but only gE-deleted vaccines were used in the herd of origin within the past 12 months
- Isolated for at least 30 days and tested after 21 days, where all pigs in isolation must be negative in the test

Criteria for approval of free status for country or zone
- The disease must be notifiable
- Epidemiological evidence for absence of virus
- Serological surveillance implemented
- No evidence and all serological tests negative for at least 12 months
- Control and recording of animal movement must have been adequate to ensure that recontamination of clear areas has not occurred
- Clear plans for monitoring of the disease in future

Criteria for approval of an eradication programme against AD
- The disease must be notifiable
- Participation in the programme must be compulsory
- Serological test scheme involves all herds (sampling at holding or at slaughterhouse)
- Where positive results are found, the herd must be restricted and not released until a negative test has been obtained at least 21 days after removal of the last positive animal
- Control and recording of animal movement must be sufficient to allow effective epidemiological investigations
- Vaccine in use must be gE-deleted
- Diagnostic tests must meet European standards

2.4.2.2. Trade regulations for IBR

Under Decision 93/42/EEC countries have for the first time been approved as free from IBR, and in 1995 official eradication programmes for IBR in Austria and Sweden were approved by the EC. By Commission Decision of 29 March 1995 concerning additional guarantees relating to IBR for cattle destined for certain parts of the territory of the Community, trade regulations for IBR were established in the EU. In Decision 2004/215/EC additional guarantees apply to countries in Annex I under 64/432/ECC Art.9 (approved eradication programme) and in Annex II under 64/432/ECC Art.10 (free from disease). So far, Germany is listed in Annex I of Decision 2004/558/EC and Denmark, Austria, Sweden, Finland, as well as the region Bolzano in Italy are mentioned in Annex II.

Switzerland and Norway were also recognised as free from IBR in the Bilateral Agreements (Decision 2004/78/EC). Additional measures were provided in Decision 2004/558/EC to ensure that the objectives of Art.9 of Directive 64/432/EEC are being met, with limited implications for trade (Anonymous, 2005a).

The conditions for recognising of freedom from disease and maintenance of the status strictly follow the OIE code. The conditions for trade were subdivided according to the purpose of the cattle traded: animals for breeding purposes, and animals for immediate slaughter. In the context of the present thesis, only the conditions regarding breeding animals will be examined. The movement of cattle to areas of equal health status is possible without further requirements.

Transfer to free areas
- No clinical or pathological signs of IBR for at least 12 months in herd of origin
- Quarantine station for 30 days prior to shipment
- All quarantined animals negative in serological test not earlier than 21 days after arrival at quarantine
- Test for antibodies against entire BoHV-1 or against gB
- Not vaccinated

Transfer to areas where an approved eradication programme is in operation
- No clinical or pathological signs of IBR for at least 12 months in herd of origin
- Quarantine station for 30 days prior to shipment
- All quarantined animals negative in serological test not earlier than 21 days after arrival at quarantine
- Vaccinated animals: Test for gE-Antibodies
- Non-vaccinated animals: Test for antibodies against entire BoHV-1 or against gB

In December 2005, the Animal Health and Welfare Panel (AHAW) of the European food safety association (EFSA) published, on behalf of the European Commission (EC), a scientific opinion on the definition of a BoHV-1 free animal and herd and described the requirements needed to obtain recognition of herd freedom. Furthermore, the role of vaccination and the probability of release of the virus into free holdings, following the adoption of Commission Decision 2004/558/EC were discussed. Based on this report, conclusions were drawn and recommendations made as issued in the opinion (Anonymous, 2005a, Anonymous, 2005b). The following definitions were suggested by the EFSA, expecting the EU to adopt them in near future.

BoHV-1 free animal
- Showing no clinical signs of IBR
- Subjected to a specific protocol* that assures sufficient probability (99.98%) that it is not infected
  OR
  originating from a BoHV-1 free herd in a BoHV-1 free zone where the surveillance programme assures sufficient probability (99.8% **) that herds are not infected

It was stated that the free status of an animal may be ascertained more accurately if it has not been vaccinated because non-vaccinated cattle can be tested by the more sensitive gB-blocking ELISA (Anonymous, 2005a).

BoHV-1 free herd
• All infected animals have been removed • Biosecurity measures are applied that prevent introduction of BoHV-1 by any means • Subjected to a specific protocol* assuring sufficient probability that infection is not present **OR** is located in a free zone, where the applied surveillance programme assures sufficient probability (99.8% **) that herds are not infected

* A protocol includes reference to repeat testing, vaccination, status of herd/zone, quarantine, etc and also the time period of "freedom" from BoHV-1
** Based on the calculations for a free zone / country

2.4.3. Import regulations of Switzerland

Under Bilateral Agreement I of 1 July 2002, Switzerland is subject to the trade regulations of the European Union (Decision 2004/78/EC). Before, other bilateral veterinary agreements such as the Agricultural Agreement of 21 June 1999 had already facilitated European trade with animals and their products. However, only the adoption of the Bilateral Agreement clearly established the equal status of Norway, Switzerland, and the EU member states regard to animal diseases. On 9 of December 2004, resolutions on the trade of agricultural goods based on Bilateral Agreement I were adopted by the Mixed Veterinary Committee of the EU and its neighbouring states within the scope of Commission Decision 2005/22/EC.

Switzerland itself has adopted new import regulations for cattle effective 1 July 2004 and for pigs effective 1 March 2005 regarding the import from EU member states and Norway. But due to the high animal health standard in Switzerland, many additional guarantees may be requested from the exporting country and SFVO publishes lists of countries from which no additional guarantees are required because they are officially free from the respective diseases, namely AD, IBR, bovine leukosis and *Brucella melitensis*. Technical guidelines for the Cantonal veterinary offices issued by SFVO recommend further measures to monitor imported animals after import. But the legal basis for implementing such measures is provided by Cantonal law and is in the legislative competence of the Cantons.

It is worth mentioning that the regulations and agreements do not only deal with animal diseases and health standards but also with animal welfare issues like transport conditions and traceability of live animals by clear and equivalent identification practices. In the present thesis, only the conditions concerning animal health are considered.

2.4.3.1. Import regulations for pigs

For the importation of pigs, the additional guarantees granted by the exporting country under EU Directive Art.9 concern AD, transmissible gastroenteritis, and *Brucella suis* infection. Pursuant to Art.10, freedom from diseases notifiable to the EU listed in Annex E, Part I, of 64/432/EEC must be guaranteed in any case for European trade and includes CSF, African swine fever, rabies, brucellosis, FMD, Anthrax, and swine vesicular disease.

Based on the Agricultural Agreement of 1999, Annex 11, and the Bilateral Agreements, the new import regulations for pigs were implemented on 1 March 2005. Figure 5 provides an overview of the import process for live pigs.

Import of live pigs from EU member states and Norway

- Imports must be registered by the importer in advance with the Cantonal veterinarian of the respective Canton:
  - place of separation must be specified
  - Cantonal veterinarian decides on separation conditions and duration
  - arrival of the animals must be notified to the cantonal veterinarian within 24 hours by the importer
- Required documents:
  - general import license from Federal Agricultural Office
  - health certificate consistent with 64/432/EEC or electronic certificate in TRACES for each separation facility
  - certificate assures that conditions are fulfilled according to Agricultural Agreement of
    1999, Annex 11, App. 2
  - certificate assures that animals were not vaccinated against EP/APP and PRRS according to legislation on animal diseases
- At the border, only documents are checked, physical examination only on suspicion of irregularities
- Transport conditions consistent with animal protection legislation
- Direct transport to separation facility
- Cantonal veterinarian decides on separation instructions on the basis of technical guidelines

Technical guidelines for separation for Cantonal veterinarians

- Imported animals must be separated and subjected to EP / APP sanitation measures
- Separation facility is assigned by the importer and accepted by the Cantonal veterinarian if it fulfils the condition of an EP separation facility according to Art. 245f of legislation on animal diseases
- No contact with other pigs, personnel is banned from other pig establishments
- Animals and sentinel pigs have not been medicated within the last three weeks
- Cantonal veterinarian designates responsible veterinarian for monitoring, duration of separation and examinations needed
- Responsible veterinarian is responsible for clinical surveillance, blood sampling and compliance with separation instructions
- If there is a case of notifiable disease, Cantonal veterinarian decides on culling of the animal or of all the animals
- Examinations and measures in separation:
  - serological examination for APP and PRSS when all pigs are three months old
  - if all results are negative, ten sentinel pigs (between 10 weeks and 6 months of age, serologically negative to APP) are exposed to the imported animals in close contact
  - after four weeks, second blood sampling in imported and sentinel pigs for serological examination for APP and PRSS
  - if vaccination is suspected in an animal, it must be slaughtered immediately
  - sentinel animals are subjected to direct slaughtering
  - when all pigs are nine months old, treatment against mycoplasma for fourteen days
- Suspension of separation by decision of the Cantonal veterinarian

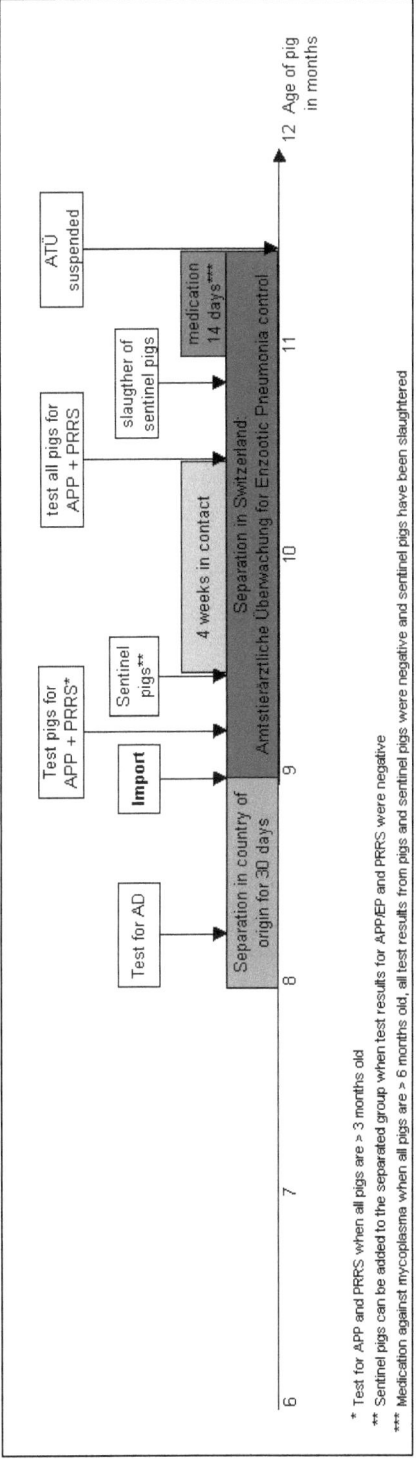

* Test for APP and PRRS when all pigs are > 3 months old
** Sentinel pigs can be added to the separated group when test results for APP/EP and PRRS were negative
*** Medication against mycoplasma when all pigs are ≥ 6 months old, all test results from pigs and sentinel pigs were negative and sentinel pigs have been slaughtered

Figure 5. Overview of the processes for importing live pigs into Switzerland from countries not free from AD according to Swiss import regulations of 1 March 2005 (described in Section 2.4.3.1; age of traded breeding pig assumed as reported by SUISAG (Swiss pig breeders association))

The required quarantine and sanitary measures for import of pigs from third countries outside EU and Norway are very strict and make an import from those countries very unlikely. In the past five years, no pigs were imported from third countries. Therefore, import regulations for third countries are not further considered in this context.

2.4.3.2. Import regulations for cattle

For cattle, the additional guarantees granted by the exporting country under EU Directive Art.9 concern only IBR. Pursuant to Art.10, freedom from diseases notifiable to the EU listed in Annex E, Part I, of 64/432/EEC must be guaranteed in any case for European trade. These include rabies, *brucella abortus*, FMD, tuberculosis, infectious bovine pleuropneumonia, Anthrax, and enzootic bovine leukosis.

Based on the Agricultural Agreement of 1999, Annex 11, and the Bilateral Agreements the new import regulations for cattle were implemented effective 1 July 2004. Figure 6 provides an overview of the import process for live cattle.

Import of live cattle from EU member states and Norway

- Imports must be registered by the importer in advance with the Cantonal veterinarian of the respective Canton:
  - Cantonal veterinarian informed about separation abroad at least one week before import
  - arrival of the animals must be notified to the Cantonal veterinarian within 24 hours by the importer
- Required documents:
  - general import license from Federal Agricultural Office
  - health certificate consistent with 64/432/EEC (Certificate F) for each separation facility or electronic certificate in TRACES
  - certificate assures that conditions are fulfilled according to Agricultural Agreement of
    1999, Annex 11, App. 2, especially the additional conditions regarding IBR
  - certificate assures that animals were not vaccinated against IBR
- Requirements in exporting country concerning IBR if country not officially free:
  - establishment: must have had no evidence of IBR for at least 12 months
  - animal: separated for 30 days and all separated animals examined serologically after at least 21 days with negative result, no vaccination against IBR
- Further requirements in exporting country:
  - establishment: must be officially free from tuberculosis, brucellosis and enzootic bovine leukosis
  - animal: examined serologically for tuberculosis, brucellosis and enzootic bovine leucosis within 30 days before shipment if country is not officially free
- Animal born after 1 June 2001
- Checking of documents and physical examination of all animals at the border
- Transport conditions consistent with animal protection legislation and no import of animals later than 250 days in gestation
- Direct transport to separation facility
- Cantonal veterinarian decides on separation instructions on the basis of technical guidelines

Technical guidelines for separation for cantonal veterinarians

- Imported animals must be separated
- Separation facility is assigned by the importer and must prevent contact with domestic cattle (5m distance on pasture, double fenced, separated indoor areas)
- Where no separation is possible, contact animals are under movement ban and would be included in any actions taken after incident (e.g. stamping out)
- Cantonal veterinarian designated responsible veterinarian for monitoring, duration of separation and necessary examinations depending on current risk situation
- Responsible veterinarian is responsible for clinical surveillance, blood sampling and compliance with separation instructions and visits the establishment at least once
- Only staff and officials are allowed into the stable (emergencies exempted) and they are obliged to change clothes and disinfect shoes and hands before contact with other cattle
- If there is a case of notifiable disease, Cantonal veterinarian decides on treatment or culling and all medical treatment requires official permission
- Ear tags have to be exchanged under supervision of the responsible veterinarian within 21 days after import
- Examinations and measures in separation:
  - all animals from IBR-free countries: separation suspended after exchange of earmarks
  - at least one animal from non-IBR-free country: blood sampling after 21 days, serological examination for IBR (and brucellosis if country not free) and separation suspended by Cantonal veterinarian if all results negative
- If separated group contained less than seven animals:
  - destination herd is put under movement ban for three weeks
  - three to ten weeks after suspension of movement ban, a control sample for IBR from seven contact animals must be taken (but not from the imported animal)
- If separated group contains seven or more animals:
  separation suspended, no further measures in destination herd

The required quarantine and sanitary measures for import of cattle from countries outside EU and Norway are very strict and make an import from these countries very unlikely. In the last five years, no cattle were imported from third countries. Therefore, import regulations for third countries are not further considered in this context.

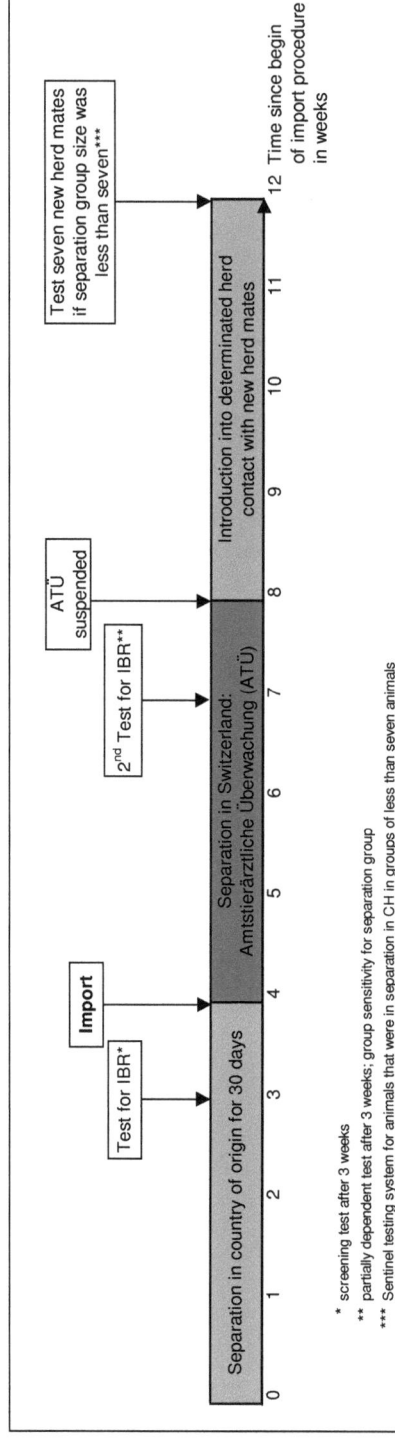

Figure 6. Overview of the processes for importing live cattle into Switzerland from countries not free from IBR according to Swiss import regulation of 1 July 2004 (Section 2.4.3.2).

2.5. RISK ANALYSIS FOR INTERNATIONAL TRADE

The principal aim of import risk analysis is to provide importing countries with an objective and defensible method of assessing the risk associated with the importation of animals, animal products, animal genetic material, feedstuffs, virological products and pathological material. It is a relatively new and evolving discipline, gaining more and more impact in international trade (Vose, 1997).

In the context of import risk analysis the term 'risk analysis' refers to a process, which embraces a series of steps from hazard identification, through qualitative or quantitative assessments of risk, to the resultant management decisions. Risk assessment as part of the risk analysis process proved to be a valuable method to support decision-makers regarding complex situations (Hathaway, 1991). It is a powerful tool to help them to a better understanding of the faced risks, the effectiveness of risk management strategies and of the value of further research to reduce any uncertainty in the model (Vose, 1997).

The term 'risk assessment' refers to the process of estimating the probability and impact of a particular hazard within the process of risk analysis. The OIE adopted the model and terminology first described by Covello and Merkhofer (1993) for risk assessment which is designed to assess the actual magnitude of the risk for specified consequences in a given situation. It can then be used to decide whether the risk is acceptable as it stands, or whether sanitary measures are required (Anonymous, 2004c). There are qualitative and quantitative approaches to risk assessment. In most cases, a qualitative assessment is conducted first. Only if a significant risk is demonstrated and the qualitative estimate is not sufficient for decision making, a quantitative assessment follows. The reliability of the quantitative assessment strongly depends on availability and sufficient quality of data.

According to the document "Basic Principles for Risk Analyses conducted at the SFVO", the risk analysis process is structured only into the three elements risk management, risk assessment and risk communication while hazard identification is seen as a part of risk assessment (Breidenbach et al., 2004; Anonymous, 2002). Therefore the present thesis represents a complete risk assessment according to the principles of SFVO while risk management and risk communication lies in the responsibility of other departments at the SFVO.

Chapter 3   Material & Methods

3.1.   RISK ASSESSMENT

All the steps undertaken in the present project were part of the risk assessment process. Detailed description of the different components are given below.

Two separated risk assessments following the OIE code, Part I, section 1.3. on risk analysis (Anonymous, 2005e) were conducted regarding the import of marker-vaccinated pigs and cattle, respectively. Despite the multiple analogies between the two herpesviruses causing AD and IBR, there exist some important differences in trade and management of the two livestock species. Furthermore, the divergent import regulations and recommendations for international trade made it inevitable to conduct two separate assessments. Therefore, the definitions for the risk assessment processes such as detailed risk profile and assumptions are provided in the model descriptions for AD and IBR, respectively.

As outlined in the principles for risk analysis by SFVO, current information was collected, documented and evaluated according to scientific criteria by means of literature research and expert elicitations. Existing knowledge gaps, limitations and uncertainties were transparently documented. As required for a quantitative risk assessment, the result is expressed as a numerical value on the basis of mathematical models (Breidenbach et al., 2004; Anonymous, 2002). This allowed for quantitative comparison of different risk pathways, implementing diverse sanitary measures.

3.2.   SCENARIO TREES

As a first step, in order to provide a conceptual framework of the biological pathways associated with the hypothetical import of marker-vaccinated live cattle and pigs, scenario trees were developed for both diseases (Figures 7-10 and 12-15). The intention was to assist in conveying the range and types of pathways considered in a simple, transparent and meaningful fashion. The trees are a graphical depiction to identify pathways, information requirements, to ensure a logical chain of events in space and time, and to clarify ideas and understanding of the problem. Furthermore, they provided the framework for the development of the quantitative models. By convention, events were described in boxes, while the probability of an event was described by a line emanating from the respective box (Anonymous, 2004c). These scenario trees have a similar structure as decision trees, except that all nodes are probability nodes and have a value associated with them.

3.3. LITERATURE RESEARCH AND ELICITING EXPERT OPINION

Input data for the different nodes identified in the scenario trees was found by searching literature. However, not for all nodes reliable values could be found.

In complete absence of data, or if the existing data is scarce or might not be representative, an approach utilising expert opinion is recommended. To avoid problems with contrary estimates from different experts and to add a literature base to the estimates, we provided the expert group some days before the meetings with an estimate drawn from literature data, where data existed. We chose Pert distributions for most values, as the terms minimum, maximum, and most likely were easy to explain to experts not familiar with modelling and probability distributions. At the expert group meetings, the suggested input values were discussed in plenum until a consensus was found. The output reflected combined literature and expert opinion based values.

The group consisted of three experts from the fields of virology, epidemiology and risk assessment. In a first meeting with the expert group in February 2005, the scenario tree for AD was discussed and refined. Throughout the whole process of risk assessment, the scenario tree was subjected to refinements and changes. The second scenario tree regarding IBR was discussed and refined at the 4th expert meeting in March 2006.

After starting with literature research, the first suggestions for input values for AD were presented at the 2nd expert meeting in June 2005. Literature was found searching PubMed for different keywords, and finally, input values have been validated by the expert group at 3rd expert meeting in December 2005. A first draft for the AD model was presented at the 4th expert meeting in March 2006. Literature concerning IBR was also collected already from the start of the project, but input values were not defined before December 2005 and first presented at the 4th expert meeting.

3.4. MODEL AND SOFTWARE

Two stochastic models using Monte Carlo sampling for simulation in a Microsoft Excel spreadsheet were developed for both AD and IBR. The models were structured as suggested within the course "Evaluation of complex surveillance systems" (Martin and Cameron, 2006; Cameron and Martin, 2003). As an overview, Tables IV and XII show all nodes and their possible outcomes in one table.

The spreadsheet was composed of two worksheets. One contained the scenario tree in a Microsoft Excel version and the other all input values, calculations, and outputs of the model. In the latter, values were ordered by type of node, starting with outputs, then all inputs for infection nodes, followed by detection nodes and category nodes. Further calculations and submodels are presented in additional worksheets.

The stochastic models used for the risk assessment were developed using @RISK for Excel provided by Palisade Corporation, Ithaca, New York, USA.

@RISK is a Microsoft Excel add-in that uses Monte Carlo simulation technique to show quantitative and graphical results for all possible outcomes of a model. Uncertain values are represented by @RISK functions to include a range of possible values and the result is presented as distributions of possible outcomes and the probabilities of them occurring.

Both models were run with 10^6 iterations to provide stable results.

3.5. MODEL FOR AUJESZKY'S DISEASE

3.5.1. Risk profile

3.5.1.1. Aim of model and assessment

The aim of the risk assessment was to estimate the probability of introduction of AD into Switzerland through import of a live domestic pig (*Sus scrofa domesticus*) vaccinated with an AD marker vaccine and transmission of the virus to a Swiss herd mate at any point in the life of the pig. Pigs for immediate slaughter were not within the scope of this assessment. There was no consequence assessment done because the infection of one single pig of the national herd is seen as an unacceptable outcome in all scenarios.

The model was built to derive a quantitative estimate as outcome for the risk assessment regarding the problem defined above. The estimate of the probability of introduction into Swiss national herd through import of a vaccinated animal is compared with the probability through import of a non-vaccinated animal imported from countries not free from AD.

3.5.1.2. Possible hazards

Possible hazards were imported swine vaccinated with a marker vaccine against AD but latently infected. This applied to live pigs from countries not free from AD where marker vaccination was practiced.

3.5.1.3. Endangered values

Sufferers in case of an incident

In general, Swiss economy (lost of export advantages), veterinary service (costs of a new eradication programme), game wardens and hunters (controlling, surveillance and eradication in corresponding wildlife population) would be affected. Particularly, for Swiss pig farmers, pet and livestock owners of other species also susceptible to AD like livestock (cattle, sheep etc.) or carnivore pets (dogs, cats), and the Swiss wild boar population, the effects would be serious.

AD has no potential of zoonosis so there is no danger for human health.

Gainers from no incident

Swiss producers (augmented access to foreign breeding stock, continuing export advantages) and European producers (high quality standards in pigs exported from Switzerland) profit from Switzerland's freedom from AD and would benefit from less restrictive import regulations (access to genetics, augmented trade).

3.5.1.4. Assumptions

Several assumptions were made to construct a model applicable to different countries. We decided that only herds with officially free status qualify for export of pigs to Switzerland. This applied to vaccinated and non-vaccinated herds. The possibility of exporting vaccinated animals was only considered in the context of an official eradication programme approved by the EU Commission. Despite some variations, requirements for the vaccination scheme were at least two vaccinations between 10 and 14 weeks of age and boostering three times a year in breeding animals all over Europe.

3.5.2. Scenario tree

3.5.2.1. Release assessment Aujeszky's disease

As explained in section 3.2, a scenario tree was drawn for the process of importing a pig into Switzerland. The release assessment describes the steps from selecting a pig for import until the animal reaches the border and is shown in Figures 7 and 8. Therefore, it provides the probability that PRV would be carried into Switzerland by one single imported pig.

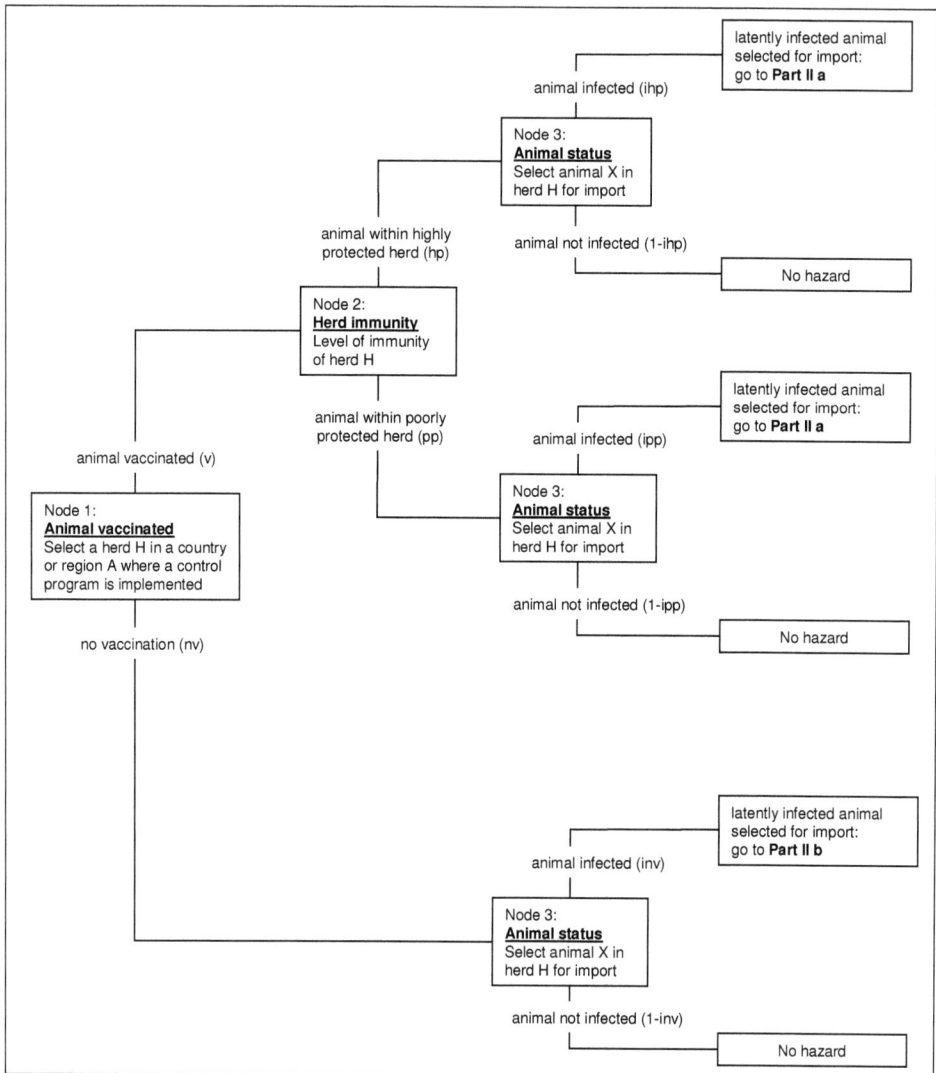

Figure 7. Release assessment for AD, Part I: Selection of animal

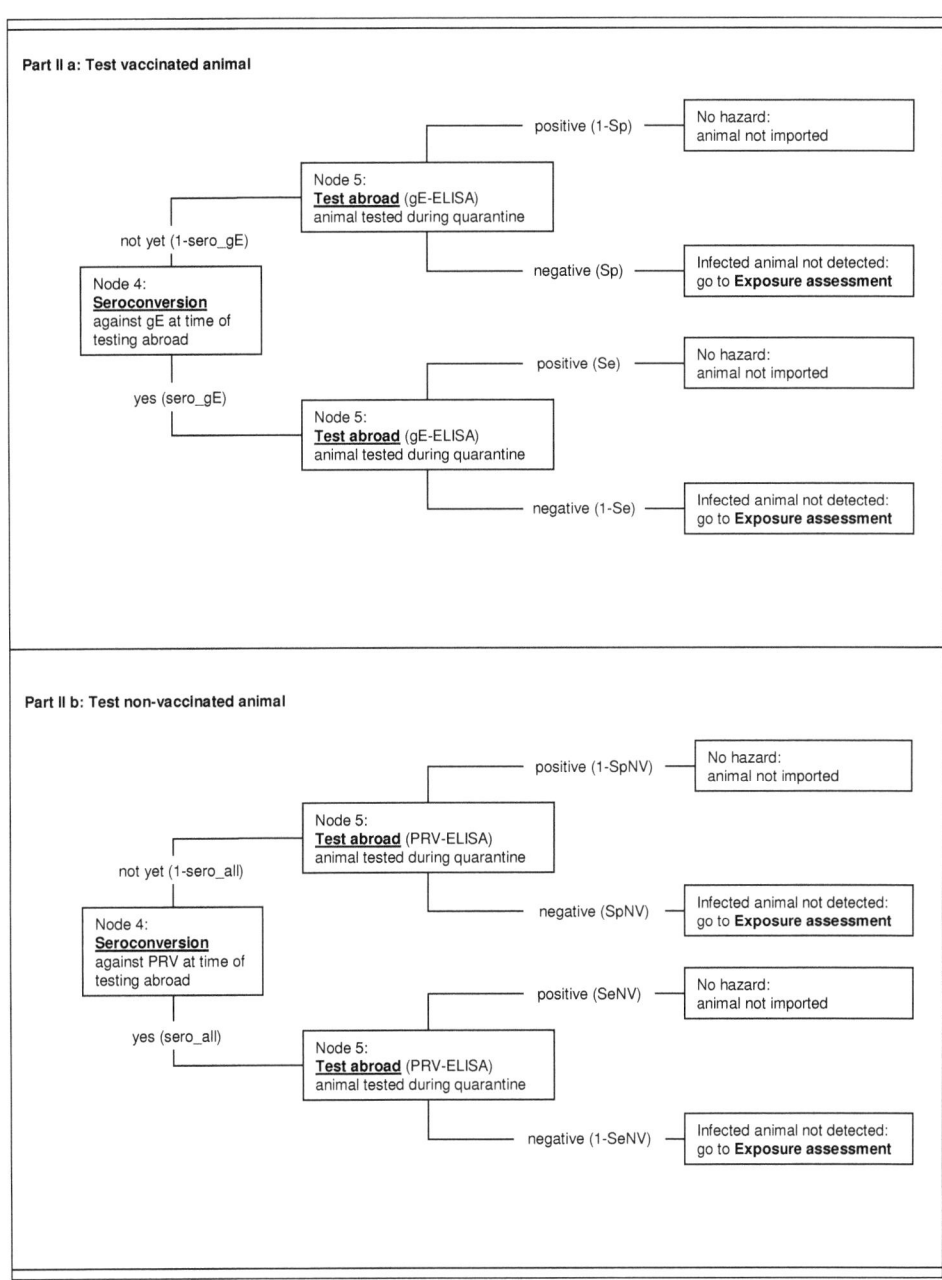

Figure 8. Release assessment for AD, Part II: Quarantine and test abroad

3.5.2.2. Exposure assessment Aujeszky's disease

The exposure assessment describes the steps from arrival in Switzerland until introduction into domestic herd and subsequent infection of a domestic pig. Therefore, it provides the probability that a domestic pig would get infected if a latently infected animal was imported as shown in Figures 9 and 10. It was divided into two parts, separation in Switzerland and introduction into domestic herd.

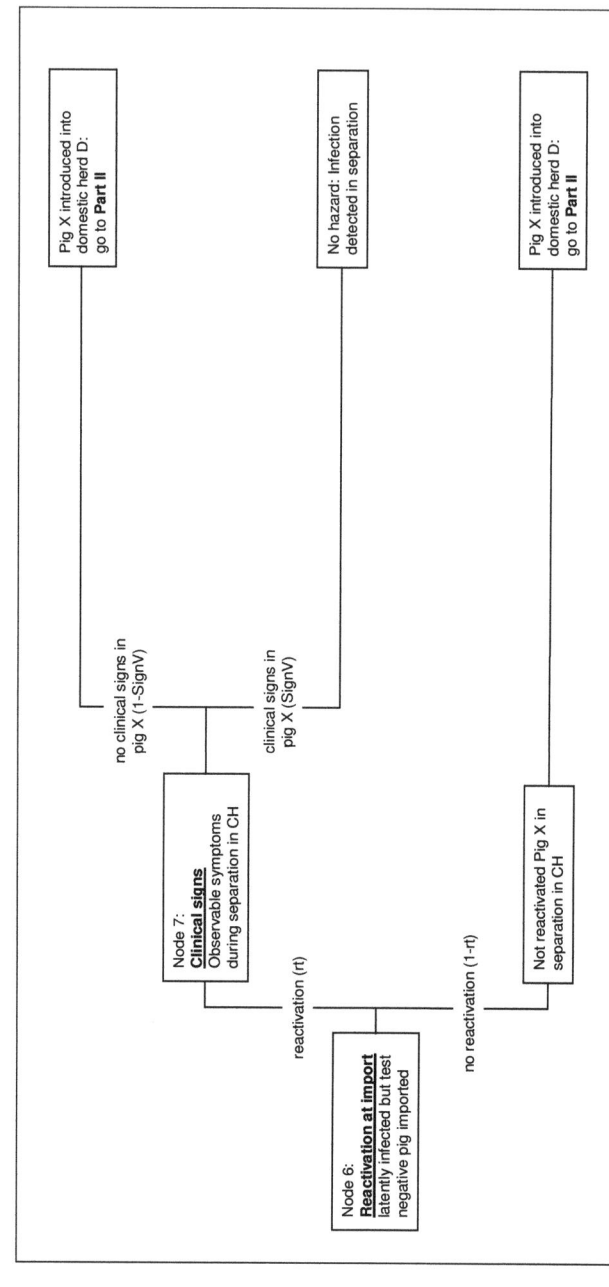

Figure 9. Exposure assessment for AD, Part I: Separation in Switzerland

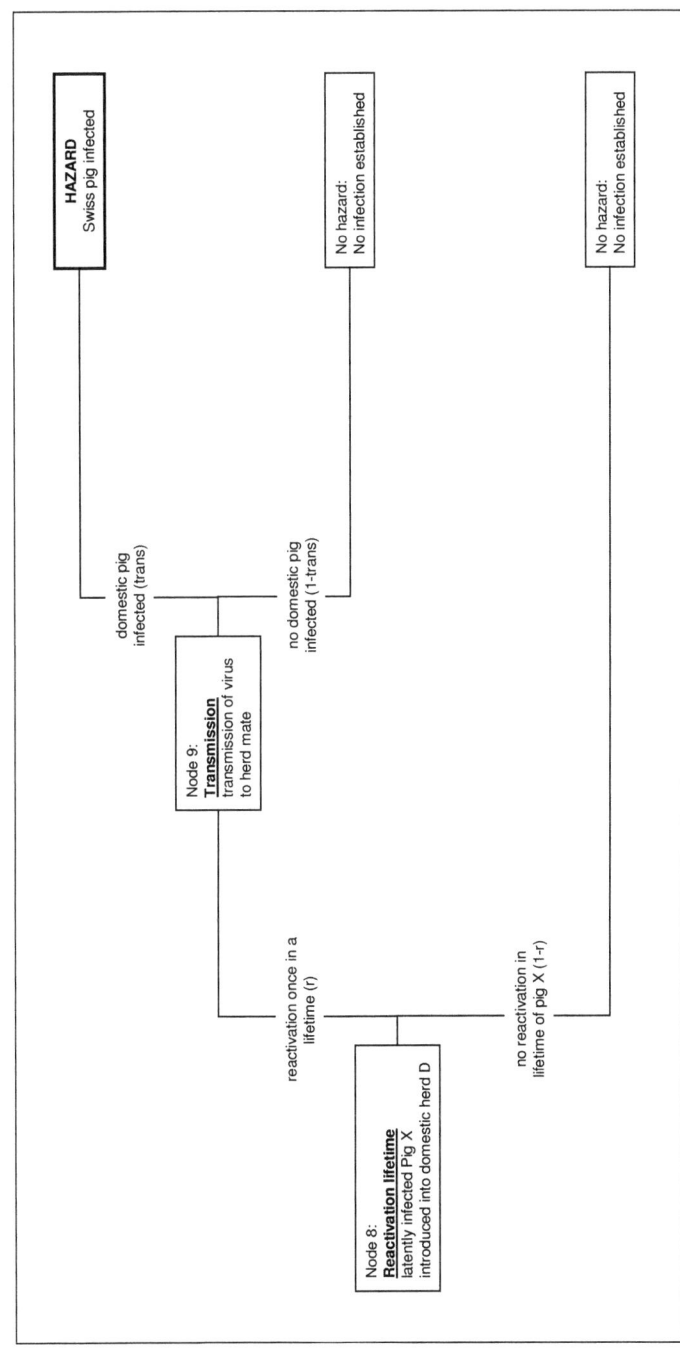

Figure 10. Exposure assessment for AD, Part II: Introduction into domestic herd

3.5.3. Overview and used parameters

In Table IV an overview over the modelled processes and a summary of the different steps within the model is given. The input parameters and abbreviations are defined in Table V.

Table IV. Model overview for Aujeszky's disease

Model Aujeszky's disease

Node	Name	Type	Outcome	Next Node	Data source
1	Animal vaccinated	Category risk	Yes No	2 3	Input
2	Herd immunity	Category risk	highly protected poorly protected	3 3	Estimate based on literature and expert opinion
3	Animal status	Infection	Infected Not infected	4 No hazard	Submodel herd prevalence + estimate for inherd-prevalence based on literature and expert opinion
4	Seroconversion	Category detection	Yes Not yet	5 6	Estimate based on literature and expert opinion
5	Test abroad	Detection	negative positive	6 No hazard	Bayes model for Sensitivity and Specificity
6	Reactivation at import	Category detection	Yes No	7 8	Estimate based on literature and expert opinion
7	Clinical signs	Detection	No Yes	8 No hazard	Estimate based on literature and expert opinion
8	Reactivation lifetime	Category risk	Yes No	9 No hazard	Estimate based on expert opinion
9	Transmission	Category risk	Yes No	**Hazard** No hazard	Estimate based on literature and expert opinion

Submodel herd prevalence

Node	Name	Outcome	Next Node	Data source
3a 1)	Herd infection status	Herd infected Herd not infected	3a 2) 3a 3)	True prevalence calculated based on data from exporting country
3a 2)	First qualifying test	negative positive	3a 4) not qualified	(= false negatives)
3a 3)	Time until next test	new infected not new infected	3a 4) 3a 5)	Incidence data from exporting country converted for test frequency
3a 4)	Second qualifying test	negative positive	3a 6) not qualified	(= false negatives)
3a 5)	Time until next test	new infected not new infected	3a 6) 3a 7)	
3a 6)	Third qualifying test	negative positive	**Hazard** not qualified	(= false negatives)
3a 7)	Time until next test	new infected not new infected	**Hazard** No hazard	(= new infected between third test and export)

Table V. Definitions of parameters used in the AD model

Nr.	Node	Name	Description
1	Animal vaccinated	v	Proportion of vaccinated imported animals
		nv	Proportion of imported non-vaccinated animals
2	Herd immunity	hp	Proportion of highly protected vaccinated herds
		pp	Proportion of poorly protected vaccianted herds
3	Animal status	ihp	Probability of infection in a vaccinated animal from a highly protected herd
		ipp	Probability of infection in a vaccinated animal from a poorly protected herd
		inv	Probability of infection in a non-vaccinated animal
		Inherdprev_hp	Proportion of infected animals within a highly protected vaccinated herd if infected
		Inherdprev_pp	Proportion of infected animals within a poorly protected vaccinated herd if infected
		Inherdprev_nv	Proportion of infected animals within a non-vaccinated herd
		HPrev	Estimated proportion of infected vaccinated herds within herds certified as free from infection
		HPrev_nv	Estimated proportion of infected non-vaccinated herds within herds certified as free from infection
		TP	True herd level prevalence derived from apparent prevalence
		HSENS	Herd level sensitivity of the country's surveillance programme
		HSPEC	Herd level specificity of the country's surveillance programme
		Prev	Proportion of infected herds as reported by the country's authorities
		Inc	Number of newly infected herds per year as reported by the country's authorities
		Inc4	Incidence rate for a four months period
		HPrevMean	Mean proportion of infected vaccinated herds within herds certified as free from infection
		HPrevMean_nv	Mean proportion of infected non-vaccinated herds within herds certified as free from infection
4	Seroconversion	age	Age of the imported animal at time of import
		conv_gE	Number of days until seroconversion against gE after infection in a vaccinated animal
		conv_all	Number of days until seroconversion against gB after infection in a non-vaccinated animal
		sero_gE	Probability that a vaccinated animal has seroconverted at time of testing abroad
		sero_all	Probability that a non-vaccinated animal has seroconverted at time of testing abroad

Nr.	Node	Name	Description
5	Test abroad	Se	Sensitivity of gE-blocking ELISA for vaccinated animals
		Sp	Specificity of gE-blocking ELISA for vaccinated animals
		SeNV	Sensitivity of PRV ELISA for non-vaccinated animals
		SpNV	Specificity of PRV ELISA for non-vaccinated animals
6	Reactivation at import	rt	Probability of reactivation at time of import in a vaccinated animal
		rtNV	Probability of reactivation at time of import in a non-vaccinated animal
7	Clinical signs	SignV	Probability of clinical signs in a vaccinated animal after reactivation of latent infection
		SignNV	Probability of clinical signs in a non-vaccinated animal after reactivation of latent infection
8	Reactivation lifetime	r	Probability of reactivation once in the lifetime of the imported animal
9	Transmission	trans	Probability of virus transmission to naiv contact animal from a vaccinated animal once latent infection is reactivated
		transNV	Probability of virus transmission to contact animal from a non-vaccinated animal once latent infection is reactivated

3.5.4. Input values and calculations

The described model represents the import of one single pig from the example region Spain. Spain was chosen because there, AD was endemic and an eradication programme approved by the EU Commission using marker-vaccination as a possible measure was in operation. Therefore, reports with data on the programme design as well as on disease occurrence were available.

3.5.4.1. Node 1: Animal vaccinated (Input value)

The proportion of animals that are vaccinated (**v**) was fixed at 1 to model import of vaccinated animals. For comparison, **v** could be fixed at 0 to model import of non-vaccinated animals because $nv = 1 - v$.

3.5.4.2. Node 2: Herd immunity (Input value)

We estimated the proportion of herds that are likely to reach a high herd level immunity (**hp**) through vaccination and therefore would only have low inherd prevalence levels once the virus is introduced. By contrast, in poorly protected herds (**pp**) major outbreaks would occur resulting in high inherd prevalences, as immunity of the majority of pigs was not sufficient to prevent infection and spread.

We defined a minor outbreak as an outbreak where inherd prevalences did not reach more than 40%. Assuming well-protected animals only cause minor outbreaks after infection, resulting inherd prevalence after infection in those herds is below 40%. Other outbreaks were thought to be major and lead to higher inherd prevalences.

Parameters were derived from literature data. Leontides et al. (1995) found 34% of 79 farrow-to-finish and 54% of 170 farrow-to-feeder units having prevalences below 20%, but they only sampled breeding pigs within those herds. Maes et al. (2000) reported 32% of 115 herds having inherd prevalences below 20%.

Therefore we used a PERT DISTRIBUTION with the following values for the probability of a vaccinated herd being highly protected (**hp**):

Minimum 11%
Most likely 32%
Maximum 54%   (where $pp = 1 - hp$)

3.5.4.3. Node 3: Animal status (Calculation)

The probability of infection of the imported animal (**ihp; ipp; inv**) was derived from herd prevalence among negatively tested herds (**HPrev; HPrev_nv**) and the respective inherd prevalence for highly protected (**Inherdprev_hp**), poorly protected (**Inherdprev_pp**) and non-vaccinated herds (**Inherdprev_nv**) as follows.

We multiplied the estimated prevalence of infected herds (**HPrev; HPrev_nv**) within negatively tested herds by the expected inherd prevalence. Based on differences in management, vaccination practice, type of holding, and regional pig density, we assumed two types of herds, highly and poorly protected, respectively. Depending on level of protection, virus spread and therefore expected inherd prevalences if virus is introduced were different. This reflects herds where minor or major outbreaks occur, once they are infected. The obtained values are shown in Table VI.

Table VI. Probability of infection of the animal: Values obtained by calculation

Name	Definition	Formula	5th percentile	median	95th percentile
ihp	Probability of infection for animal from highly protected herd	HPrev * Inherdprev_hp	0.03%	0.24%	0.92%
ipp	Probability of infection for animal from poorly protected herd	HPrev * Inherdprev_pp	0.15%	1.22%	3.67%
inv	Probability of infection for animal from non-vaccinated herd	HPrev_nv * Inherdprev_nv	0.000006%	0.00004%	0.01%

Inherd prevalences (Input value for node 3)

We estimated the prevalence within an infected herd for highly protected herds where only minor outbreaks occur (**Inherdprev_hp**), poorly protected herds where major outbreaks are very likely (**Inherdprev_pp**), and non-vaccinated herds (**Inherdprev_nv**) respectively.

Inherd prevalence for highly protected herd (**Inherdprev_hp**)
    Minimum 0.1%
    Most likely 20%
    Maximum 40%

Inherd prevalence for poorly protected herd (**Inherdprev_pp**)
    Minimum 40%
    Most likely 100%
    Maximum 100%

For non-vaccinated herds (**Inherdprev_nv**) the experts expected the same inherd prevalence once the herd was infected as for poorly protected herds.

Herd level prevalence (Input value for node 3 from submodel 'Herd prevalence')

Values for herd level prevalence among negatively tested herds were derived from Submodel Herd prevalence for vaccinated (**HPrev**) and non-vaccinated herds (**HPrev_nv**) as PERT DISTRIBUTIONS. See section 3.5.5.1 for further explanations. The values obtained from the submodel are listed in Table VII.

Table VII. Probability of infection of herd: Values derived from Submodel HPrev for Spain

Name	Definition	Formula	5th percentile	median	95th percentile
HPrev	Prevalence within negatively tested vaccinated herds	+ Inc	0.17%	1.36%	4.00%
HPrev_nv	Prevalence within negatively tested non-vaccinated herds	Inc = 0	0.000005%	0.00004%	0.01%

3.5.4.4. Node 4: Seroconversion at time of testing (Calculation)

The probability of seroconversion in an infected animal at time of testing abroad for vaccinated (**sero_gE**) and non-vaccinated animals (**sero_PRV**) was calculated as follows.

$$\text{sero\_gE} = 1 - (\text{conv\_gE} / \text{age})$$

$$\text{sero\_PRV} = 1 - (\text{conv\_PRV} / \text{age})$$

This formula was based on the assumption of a daily risk of infection for each day in the life of a pig that could be calculated as 1 divided by the age of the pig in days. This assumed that the risk of infection was constant for each day in the life of a pig, which is certainly untrue. But since the age of the pig at import lies within the narrow range from 6 to 10 months, we thought the assumption was reasonable.

Assuming a constant daily risk of infection allowed us to multiply the daily risk (= **1/age**) by the estimated days until seroconversion to calculate the probability of testing an animal exactly within these critical days before seroconversion and therefore missing the infection given that age is always more than the estimated days until seroconversion. In our case, as the minimum for age of the pig at time of selection for import (*age*) was 180 days, it was given. The obtained values are shown in Table VIII.

Table VIII. Probability of seroconversion: Values derived from calculation

Name	Definition	Formula	5th	median	95th
sero_gE	Probability of vaccinated animal seroconverted at time of testing if infected	*1 - (conv_gE / age)*	93%	95%	96%
sero_all	Probability of non-vaccinated animal seroconverted at time of testing if infected	*1 - (conv_PRV / age)*	95%	96%	97%

Age of the pig (Input value for node 4)

The age of the pig at time of selection for import into Switzerland (**age**) was modelled as a Pert distribution based on the information from SUISAG about the common age of traded breeding pigs. Following SUISAG breeding pigs are traded mostly before first service at the age of 6 to 7 months and would enter separation in the exporting country around this age. Pregnant gilts at the age of 9 to 10 months are also traded. Only young pregnant sows, which gave birth shortly after quarantine have been imported so far (Zurkirch, R., SUISAG, personal communication).

Input for age of pig (**age**) is the following PERT DISTRIBUTION:
>Minimum 180 days
>Most likely 285 days
>Maximum 310 days

Days until seroconversion (Input value for node 4)

The number of days until detectable seroconversion after infection was estimated as a Pert distribution for vaccinated (**conv_gE**) and non-vaccinated animals (**conv_PRV**). In experiments most animals were tested positive for gE-antibodies 2 weeks after infection, latest reported after 4 weeks (Eloit et al., 1989; van Oirschot et al., 1988c). Seroconversion against gE in vaccinated animals took a couple of days more than seroconversion in non-vaccinated animals. There was no case of no seroconversion described in literature. First antibodies were found one week after infection (van Oirschot, 1988a).

We used a PERT DISTRIBUTION for time until seroconversion after infection
for a vaccinated pig (**conv_gE**)
>Minimum 7 days
>Most likely 14 days
>Maximum 28 days

for a non-vaccinated pig (**conv_PRV**)
>Minimum 7 days
>Most likely 10 days
>Maximum 14 days

3.5.4.5. Node 5: Test abroad (Input value)

Sensitivity and specificity of the gE-ELISA (for node 5 from Bayes model)

For sensitivity and specificity of the gE-ELISA, values were derived using a Bayes model. The Bayes model described in paragraph 3.5.5.2 included data from 6 papers and a total of 814 positive and 4384 negative sera, respectively. The values derived from the Bayes model are shown in Table IX.

Table IX. Test performance of gE-ELISA: Values derived from Bayes model

Name	Definition	Formula	5th percentile	median	95th percentile
Se	Sensitivity of gE-ELISA	Bayes model	98.2%	98.9%	99.4%
Sp	Specificity of gE-ELISA	Bayes model	99.5%	99.7%	99.8%

Sensitivity and specificity of the PRV-ELISA (Input value for node 5)

The sensitivity (**SeNV**) and specificity (**SpNV**) of the ELISA for non-vaccinated animals was estimated as a Pert distribution based on the following literature. Durham et. al (1985) found a sensitivity of 0.96 (CI 0.94 - 0.98) and a specificity of 0.99 (CI 0.993 - 0.998) using 304 positive and 3447 negative sera, respectively. White et al. (1996) reported a sensitivity of 100% (CI 0.94 - 1.00) using 55 positive sera. Boelaert et al. (1999) proposed a sensitivity of 0.95 and a specificity of 0.99, and the producer of the test kit reported a sensitivity and a specificity of 0.995. Since there was no more data available, we decided to draw an estimate as a Pert distribution instead of implementing data from only two papers into the Bayes model, though the latter had been possible. But by using a Pert distribution, we could relay on additional information like information from producer and the estimate of Boelaert that could not be inserted into the Bayes model.

We used a PERT DISTRIBUTION for sensitivity and specificity of the PRV-ELISA (for non-vaccinated animals) with

>Sensitivity (**SeNV**) Minimum 94%
>   Most likely 98%
>   Maximum 100%
>Specificity (**SpNV**) Minimum 95%
>   Most likely 99%
>   Maximum 100%

3.5.4.6. Node 6: Reactivation at import (Input value)

The probability of reactivation in a latently infected animal during import for vaccinated (**rt**) and non-vaccinated animals (**rtNV**) was modelled as a Pert distribution. Transportation and crowding mean stress and might provoke a reactivation in these animals.

There were not many experiments documented on reactivation of PRV in latently infected vaccinated pigs and the used model (dexamethasone treatment) simulated a very high level of stress. Most data was from experiments with only once vaccinated pigs and therefore not really comparable to the situation in the field. Mean overall value suggested that around 65% of latently infected vaccinated pigs could be reactivated. Two studies where pigs were vaccinated twice led to virus reactivation in 25% of pigs (Ferrari et al., 2000; Schang et al., 1994; Mengeling et al., 1992; Schoenbaum et al., 1990; van Oirschot and Gielkens, 1984). Therefore, we assumed a most likely value for reactivation of 25%. Depending on transport duration and group size, we assumed that even in best case a reactivation rate of 1% would occur. After discussion with the experts, we agreed on a maximum value of 60% since pigs were all vaccinated at least twice and stress level was not very high.

Our conclusion after discussion with the experts was a PERT DISTRIBUTION for the probability of reactivation in vaccinated animals at import (**rt**) with

Minimum 1%
Most likely 25%
Maximum 60%

Non-vaccinated latently infected animals are much more likely to reactivate infection at import (**rtNV**). We estimated a PERT DISTRIBUTION with the opinion of the experts for the probability of reactivation in non-vaccinated animal at import (**rtNV**) with

Minimum 50%
Most likely 75%
Maximum 100%

3.5.4.7. Node 7: Clinical signs (Input value)

The probability of detectable clinical signs in a vaccinated animal after reactivation (**SignV**) was estimated. After import, the pig would have to pass the Swiss EP/APP sanitary programme including a separation of at least eight weeks (Anonymous, 2005d). During this time the animals were surveyed for any signs of disease. But clinical signs would only be detected if they were visible. Other symptoms as, for example, slight increase in body temperature or reduced daily weight gain would not be detected.

Vilnis et al. (1998) used the following clinical score for their experiment with 77 pigs: 0 = normal, 1 = nasal discharge, 2 = depressed, 3 = off-feed, 4 = nervous signs, 5 = moribund/dead. The mean total clinical score for non-vaccinated controls was 14.3 (SD 8.7) and the mean maximal clinical score on one day was 4.2 (SD 1.2). For IM vaccinated animals the mean total clinical score was 1.2 (SD 3) and the mean maximal clinical score on one day was 0.6 (SD 1). This data support the assumption that detectable clinical signs in a vaccinated pig are very unlikely because the vaccine was developed to prevent clinical signs and the losses due to them. But slight depression might occur in some cases and could be noticed. Other authors report clinical signs in vaccinated pigs after reactivation to be even more unlikely.

We concluded that clinical signs are very unlikely in vaccinated animals. After reactivation from latency, symptoms are even more unlikely than after new infection. But symptoms are not impossible and due to virulence of field virus strain, biological diversity, general health status of the animal and prudence of personnel we assumed that detected clinical signs occurred at maximum in 1 out of 100 latently infected vaccinated pigs after reactivation.

We used a PERT DISTRIBUTION for the probability of observed clinical signs in a vaccinated pig after reactivation (**SignV**) with

Minimum 0%
Most likely 0%
Maximum 1%

The probability of clinical signs in non-vaccinated animals after reactivation (**SignNV**) was fixed at 100% as pigs below ten months of age are most likely to show clinical signs. This was based on expert opinion and literature. For example, Van Rooji et al. (2004) found visible clinical signs in all four control animals and Vilnis et. al. (1998) reported a mean clinical score of 14.3 for six control pigs in the experiments described above.

3.5.4.8. Node 8: Reactivation lifetime (Input value)

The probability of reactivation in a latently infected animal at one point in the life of a breeding pig (**r**) was estimated at 100% following expert opinion. We assumed for the lifetime of a pig that there would always be at least once a stress factor strong enough to reactivate infection. Furthermore, in vaccinated animals, the vaccination would no longer be boostered and immunity would fade out. On the other hand, the animal might die due to any reason and therefore did not reactivate infection during lifetime, but there was no available data on the "reactivation rate" within the life of a pig. To get a biologically plausible input in absence of more precise data, we used a Uniform distribution with

Minimum 95%
Maximum 100%

3.5.4.9. Node 9: Transmission of virus (Input value)

The probability of virus transmission to a naïve herd mate once the infection was reactivated (**trans**) was estimated as a Pert distribution. Van Oirschot et al. (1988b) found that all 6 naive contact animals were infected which means a most likely value of 100%. The confidence interval of these findings was from 54% to 100%. In another experiment with once vaccinated, challenged and reactivated pigs, they found that all contact animals were infected too, but the sentinel pig of the twice vaccinated, challenged and reactivated group got not infected. This represented a transmission in 66% of cases with a confidence interval from 1% to 99% (van Oirschot, 1988b). With the experts, we agreed that the most likely value of transmission to susceptible naive animals was 100%. R_0 for non-vaccinated animals was estimated at 10 (de Jong and Kimman, 1994) so if once one domestic pig was infected a major outbreak among our naïve population would be most likely.

Probability of transmission of virus (**trans**) was modelled as a PERT DISTRIBUTION with

Minimum 54%
Most likely 100%
Maximum 100%

For a non-vaccinated pig, transmission probability (**transNV**) was 100% referring to expert opinion and the reported R_0 of 10 (de Jong and Kimman, 1994).

3.5.5. Submodels

3.5.5.1. Submodel Herd prevalence (Submodel for node 3)

To get a realistic assumption of the prevalence between officially negative herds we attempted to evaluate the country's eradication programme. One of the difficulties for this evaluation was our lack of knowledge on herd size and farming structure in the exporting country. The only information we got was the regulations for the eradication campaign and surveillance requirements. For example, in Spain a sample size to detect inherd prevalences above 5% with a level of confidence of 95% was required and testing was performed every four months. The exact sample size per herd size was outlined within the regulations. To obtain the officially free status, a herd had to be tested negative at least three times. The level of confidence of the programme can be seen as the herd level sensitivity at the respective threshold, but is obviously not the sensitivity for proving complete freedom. Values to model Pert distributions were then drawn from the matrix in the Submodel Herd prevalence for vaccinated (**HPrev**) and non-vaccinated herds (**HPrev_nv**).

The following input values were needed for Submodel Herd prevalence.

Apparent herd prevalence and herd incidence (Input value)

Apparent prevalence between herds (**Prev**) was modelled as a Beta distribution with the reported data from the country (Anonymous, 2004d). In Spain, this was 7736 infected herds within a total of 67'849 herds in the whole country in 2004.

Prev is modelled as RiskBeta(7736+1;67849-7736+1).

The apparent incidence rate (**Inc**) was modelled as a Gamma distribution. Data from Spain was 1567 new positives within 67'849 controlled herds in 2004. At the beginning of the year, 6169 herds were already infected; by the end of the year 7736 infected herds were recorded. The mean herd-years-at-risk were calculated as follows:

= ((**67849 herds - 6169 positive herds at beginning of the year**)
+ (**67849 herds - 7736 positive herds at end of the year**)) **divided by 2**

Then, **Inc** was modelled as RiskGamma(1567;((67849-6169)+(67849-7736))/2) (Thrusfield, 2005; Anonymous, 2004d). The obtained values are shown in Table X.

Table X. Submodel Herd prevalence: Apparent prevalence and incidence rate

Name	Definition	Formula	5th percentile	median	95th percentile
Prev	Apparent herd prevalence from data reported by Spanish authorities	Beta distribution	9.76%	9.94%	10.12%
Inc	Apparent incidence rate from data reported by Spanish authorities	Gamma distribution	2.47%	2.57%	2.68%

Surveillance programme in the country (Input value)

The expected herd level sensitivity (**HSENS**) and specificity (**HSPEC**) were derived from the regulations of the Spanish eradication programme. The level of confidence of such a programme can be seen as the herd level sensitivity at the named threshold. Since the same level of confidence was required for vaccinated and non-vaccinated herds, the same values applied for both. We assumed perfect specificity for both types of herds because positive test results would be retested with confirmatory tests to prove infection.

HSENS = 95%
HSPEC = 100%

True herd level prevalence (Calculation)

True herd level prevalence (**TP**) was calculated from apparent herd prevalence (**Prev**) with the following formula (Thrusfield, 2005).

$$TP = (Prev + HSPEC - 1) / (HSPEC + HSENS - 1)$$

For **HSENS** the value derived from the surveillance programme's confidence level was used and **HSPEC** is fixed at 100% as explained before. This lead to the following simplification of the formula above:

$$TP = Prev / HSENS$$

We were using the fixed parameters for calculating **TP** as an overall estimation of **HSENS**, ignoring the parameter herd size.

Incidence rate per 4 months (Calculation)

The annual incidence rate (**Inc**) was divided by three to calculate incidence rate for a four-month period (**Inc4**) (Thrusfield, 2005) because herds were retested three times per year.

Scenario tree for Submodel Herd prevalence

The scenario tree developed to derive the prevalence of infected herds in herds qualified for export can be seen in Figure 11. Qualified refers to a herd officially certified as free from AD, i.e. in Spain negative in three tests within a one year period. We attempted a retrospective approach and chose to ignore all information prior to the first out of three qualifying tests as a risk adverse decision.

The scenario tree lead to the following formulas:

not qualified
$$= TP * (1-HSENS)^3 + (1-TP) * Inc4 * (1-HSENS)^2 + (1-TP) * (1-Inc4) * Inc4 * (1-HSENS) + (1-TP) * (1-Inc4)^2 * (Inc4/2) + (1-TP) * (1-Inc4)^2 * (1-(Inc4/2))$$

qualified but infected
$$= TP * (1-HSENS)^3 + (1-TP) * Inc4 * (1-HSENS)^2 + (1-TP) * (1-Inc4) * Inc4 * (1-HSENS) + (1-TP) * (1-Inc4)^2 * (Inc4/2)$$

qualified and free
$$= (1-TP) * (1-Inc4)^2 * (1-(Inc4/2))$$

To get the prevalence of infected herds among negatively tested and therefore qualified herds, we had to divide the infected among qualified herds by all qualified herds.

HPrev = (qualified but infected) / (qualified but infected + qualified and free)

$$= (TP * (1-HSENS)^3 + (1-TP) * Inc4 * (1-HSENS)^2 + (1-TP) * (1-Inc4) * Inc4 * (1-HSENS) + (1-TP) * (1-Inc4)^2 * (Inc4/2)) / (TP * (1-HSENS)^3 + (1-TP) * Inc4 * (1-HSENS)^2 + (1-TP) * (1-Inc4) * Inc4 * (1-HSENS) + (1-TP) * (1-Inc4)^2 * (Inc4/2) + (1-TP) * (1-Inc4)2 * (1-(Inc4/2))$$

Most likely herd level prevalence for vaccinated herds (Model output)

The most likely value for **HPrev** (=**HPrevMean**) was calculated with the formula derived from Submodel Herd prevalence using the herd level sensitivity of the surveillance programme at its threshold.

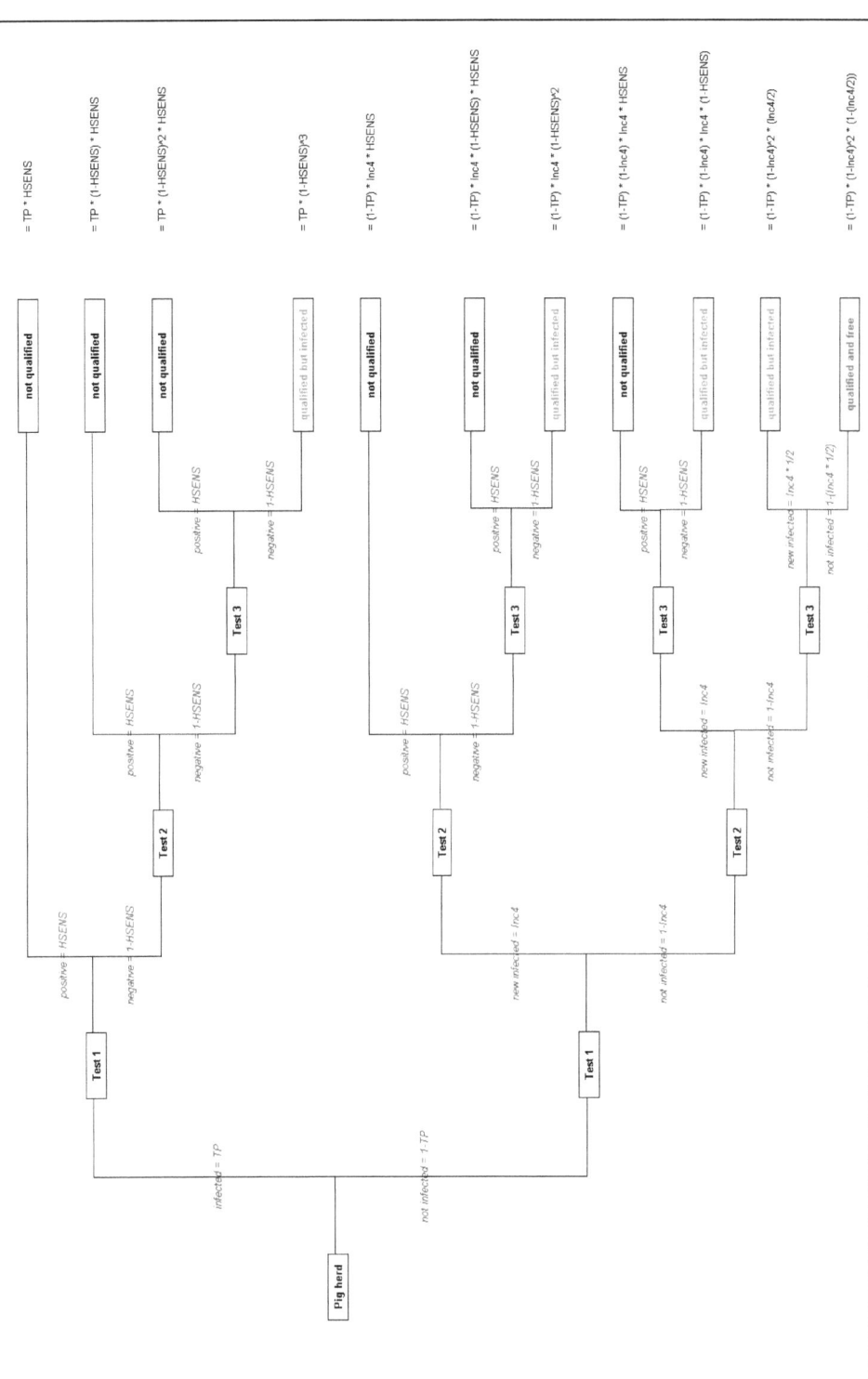

Figure 11. Submodel herd prevalence: Scenario tree for infected among negative tested herds

Minimal and maximal herd prevalence for vaccinated herds (Model output)

To estimate the possible range of the herd level prevalence we calculated **HPrev** for different herd sizes. In the Spanish regulations the sample size for variable herd sizes was given. For any herd size minimal possible prevalence if herd was not free could be calculated assuming only one infected animal in the herd (= **1 / herd size**). The minimal value for **HSENS** was calculated for herds with >1200 animals with sample size 59 and expected prevalence 0.05%. With this information, we calculated more precise estimates for **HSENS** regarding different herd sizes instead of just assuming **HSENS** as the confidence level of the surveillance programme as done for calculation of **TP** and **HPrevMean**. The intention was to get a more precise estimate for **HPrev** using the formula derived from the scenario tree with the calculated values for **HSENS** for the respective herd size as shown in Table XI in the column "plus Incidence". For single test sensitivity and specificity, we used the values derived from the Bayes model (Section 3.5.5.2) for sensitivity and specificity of gE-ELISA (Mean values 0.9783 for **Se** and 0.9971 for **Sp**).

We took into account that the reported incidence rate was only apparent, as we did not know how many of these herds had been truly newly infected and how many had just been false negatives in the last testing rounds. Therefore we repeated the calculations by assuming incidence equaled zero and all apparently newly infected herds had been false negatives in the former testing round. This is shown in Table XI in the last column "without Incidence".

The results of all calculations can be seen in the following table XI. We set the smallest value as the minimum and the greatest as the maximum value for the Pert distribution for **HPrev** (see fields with bold border).

Table XI. Submodel Herd prevalence: Expected values for HPrev for different herd sizes

Programme		Calculation		HPrev	
Herd size	Sample size	minimal inherd prev	mininal HSENS calculated	plus Incidence	without Incidence
M	n	p	HSENS		
25	all animals		= Se	0.004	0.0000002
30	26	0.033	0.61045194	0.016	0.007
40	31	0.025	0.57726251	0.018	0.009
50	35	0.020	0.54846289	0.021	0.011
70	40	0.014	0.49274462	0.026	0.015
100	45	0.010	0.43478022	0.032	0.021
200	51	0.005	0.32466607	0.048	0.035
1200	57	0.0008	0.18386624	0.076	0.060
> 1200	59	0.0005	0.17373856	0.078	0.062
as required by the spanish regulation		$= 1/M$	$= 1-(p^*(1-Se)+(1-p)^*Sp)^n$	$= Inc4+(1-HSENS)^*(Inc4+(1-HSENS)^*(Inc4+(1-HNPV)))$	$= (1-HNPV)^*(1-HSENS)^2$

Submodel Herd prevalence: Outcome for vaccinated herds (Calculation)

Based on the calculations shown above, we estimated the prevalence within negatively tested vaccinated herds (**HPrev**) as a Pert distribution with minimum 0.0000002, most likely 0.005 and maximum 0.079.

Most likely herd level prevalence in non-vaccinated herds (Model output)

For non-vaccinated herds the situation was different from vaccinated herds. In case of an introduction of virus into the herd between two testing rounds, an outbreak with clinical symptoms was very likely and the herd would not enter the next sampling round anyway.

Therefore we assumed that the incidence rate in non-vaccinated herds represented former false negatives only and we calculated the most likely value for herd level prevalence among negatively tested non-vaccinated herds (**HPrevMean_nv**) with **Inc = 0** and herd level sensitivity of the surveillance programme at its threshold (**HSENS** = confidence level of surveillance programme). The formula for **HPrevMean** then simplified for non-vaccinated herds to

$$\text{HPrevMean\_nv} = (\text{TP} * (1-\text{HSENS})^3) / (1 - \text{TP})$$

Minimal and maximal herd prevalence non-vaccinated herds (Model output)

From the result **HPrevMean** for vaccinated herds we obtained a most likely value of 0.005 and for non-vaccinated herds and for **HPrevMean_nv** a value of 0.000015. The proportion of these two values was 0.0031 (= **HPrevMean_nv** divided by **HPrevMean**) and the minimal and maximal prevalence within negatively tested non-vaccinated herds were derived by multiplication of the values for **HPrev** in vaccinated herds with this factor.

$$\text{minimal HPrev\_nv} = 0.0031 * \text{minimal HPrev}$$

$$\text{maximal HPrev\_nv} = 0.0031 * \text{maximal HPrev}$$

Submodel herd prevalence: Outcome for non-vaccinated herds (Calculation)

The most likely **HPrev_nv** was calculated as described above for Spain as 0.000015. Proportional to the **HPrev** values we estimated **HPrev_nv** as minimal 0.0000000005 and maximal 0.0002. These values were modelled as a Pert distribution.

3.5.5.2. Bayes model (Submodel for node 5)

Sensitivity (**Se**) and specificity (**Sp**) of the gE-ELISA was derived from literature data. Since 1988 several papers were published concerning the performance of the marker diagnostics for Aujeszky's disease. Following the principles of Bayes modelling, we decided to learn from the past in chronological order on the basis of a range chosen by the experts (Anonymous, 2004d).

The prior distribution for the first Bayesian update was a uniform distribution from 0.8 to 1 for sensitivity and specificity according to expert opinion. Confidence limits of the results of all experiments were within this range except for one experiment with lower specificity and it corresponded to the statements of the Veterinary Offices in France (Sens & Spec are 100%, Marechal, G., personal communication) and Germany (Sens & Spec are for sure above 0.98, Muller, T., Beer, M., Lemke, I., personal communication). This first prior was uninformed except from defining the range. A likelihood function was drawn from first experimental data and multiplied with the prior to get the first posterior. From there, after normalising the posterior, next prior and likelihood function was derived step by step through all experimental data.

Six papers were used in the model in chronological order. Not all available papers were included in the model due to different reasons. Inclusion criteria were a reasonable number of animals used in the experiment (at least more than 20) and a known test kit utilised. Two papers were excluded because there were test kits used not longer on market or there were only few animals used for the experiment. We assumed that the principles of tests were the same (all gE-blocking ELISAs); the different test kits and the animals used were comparable to each other and with the field population. There were some papers included dealing with infected animals non-vaccinated prior to challenge or animals vaccinated with gE-positive vaccines. In our model, we separated the question if antibody response rises in an infected animal (probability of seroconversion at time of testing) from detection sensitivity of the test. Our estimate for sensitivity of test was only applied to animals that did have gE-antibodies and therefore we thought experiments dealing with detecting gE antibodies in infected animals were reliable no matter if the animal was vaccinated before infection or not. Obviously, there is a biological difference in the two cases of infection. But since there was no case described in literature of a vaccinated pig that did not seroconvert against gE after field infection and time until seroconversion was already accounted for in the model, we decided to include experimental data from both types of infected animals.

Included papers:

- van Oirschot (1988b)
  experimental low dose infections, 24 sera, 22 expected positive (12 inoculated naïve pigs, 6 naïve contact animals, 4 vaccinated contact animals), 2 expected negative (vaccinated contact pigs that could not be reactivated with dexamethasone treatment)
- van Oirschot et al. (1988c)
  4542 sera, 442 expected positive (440 SPF-pigs inoculated with field virus or gE-positive vaccines, 2 vaccinated and challenged pigs), 4100 expected negative (4000 from certified free herds, 25 SPF-pigs, 25 bovine and 50 equine seras)
- Schmitt et al. (1991)
  313 sera from feral pigs, 150 expected positive, 163 expected negative (compared to latex agglutination as gold standard)
- Arias et al. (1992)
  176 sera, 74 positive (30 vaccinated and challenged, 44 challenged naïve pigs), 102 negative (55 vaccinated not challenged, 47 naïve not challenged)
- White et al. (1996)
  110 sera, all positive (pigs non-vaccinated that survived challenge infection)
- Jacobs et al. (1999)
  33 seras, 16 positive (reactors from vaccinated formerly free herds, detected by routine testing, confirmed with confirmation ELISA and PCR), 7 negative (seven uninfected non-vaccinated controls)

Excluded papers and reason for exclusion:

- Motha and Eernisse (1992)
  only 34 sera examined with Moneliffa, Suvaxyn + ClinEase ELISA
  Moneliffa (Rhone Merieux) and Suvaxyn (Duphar) test kits are not mentioned anywhere else and no longer available
- van Oirschot and Oei (1989)
  only 12 sera examined with experimental and Intervet ELISA
  Intervet test kit is no longer available (Intervet taken over by IDEXX)

From the prior distribution and the experimental data from the first paper we derived a likelihood function for the results of that experiment. This function was multiplied by the likelihood of the prior function (which, in the case of an uninformed prior, equals one) to get the posterior distribution. The posterior distribution was normalised and then used as the prior likelihood for the next experimental results to be included in the model and so on.

Finally, sensitivity and specificity was modelled as a generalised probability distribution based on the chosen range and the final normalised posterior distribution used as its underlaying density curve (Anonymous, 2004d).

The resulting mean values for sensitivity (**Se**) and specificity (**Sp**) were 0.98897 and 0.99726, respectively. The range of the values was 0.969 - 0.998 and 0.993 - 0.999.

3.6. MODEL FOR INFECTIOUS BOVINE RHINOTRACHEITIS

3.6.1. Risk profile

3.6.1.1. Aim of model and assessment

The aim of the risk assessment was to estimate the probability of introduction of IBR into Switzerland through import of live cattle (*Bos bovis*) vaccinated with an IBR marker vaccine and transmission of virus to a Swiss herd mate at any point in the life of the cattle. Cattle imported for immediate slaughter was not within the scope of this assessment. There was no consequence assessment done because the infection of one single animal of the national herd was already seen as an unacceptable outcome. The infection of sentinel animals in the determined Swiss herd, which, in fact, are part of the national herd, was not seen as introduction of disease since these animals would be under surveillance and their establishment under movement ban at this stage of the import process.

With the present model we aimed to derive a quantitative estimate regarding the question above. The estimate of the probability of introduction of IBR into the Swiss national herd through vaccinated animals was compared with the current probability through non-vaccinated animals imported from countries not free from IBR.

3.6.1.2. Possible hazards

Imported livestock vaccinated with a marker vaccine against IBR was identified as possible hazard. This applied to live cattle from countries not free from IBR where marker vaccination was practiced.

3.6.1.3. Endangered values

Sufferers in case of an incident

In general, Swiss economy (loose of export advantages and additional guarantees for imported animals) and Federal veterinary service (costs of a new eradication program) would be affected. Particularly, for Swiss cattle farmers, the effects would be serious concerning the losses through disease and eradication.

IBR has no potential of zoonosis; there is no danger for human health.

Gainers from no incident

Swiss producers (augmented access to foreign breeding stock, continuing export advantages) profit from Switzerland's freedom from IBR, whereas Swiss and European producers (augmented import to Switzerland) would benefit from less restrictive import regulations (access to genetics, augmented trade).

3.6.1.4. Assumptions

Several assumptions were made to construct a model applicable to different countries. Only herds with officially free status were seen as qualified for export of cattle to Switzerland. This applied for vaccinated and non-vaccinated herds. The possibility of exporting vaccinated animals was only seen in the context of an official eradication programme approved by the EU Commission. We assumed that the exporting country used the gB-ELISA for testing of non-vaccinated animals as recommended by EFSA (Anonymous, 2005b).

3.6.2. Scenario tree

3.6.2.1. Release assessment

As explained in section 3.2, a scenario tree was drawn for the process of importing one cattle into Switzerland. The release assessment describes the steps from selecting an animal for import until the animal reaches the boarder and is shown in Figures 12 and 13. It provides the probability that BoHV-1 would be carried into Switzerland by one single imported cattle.

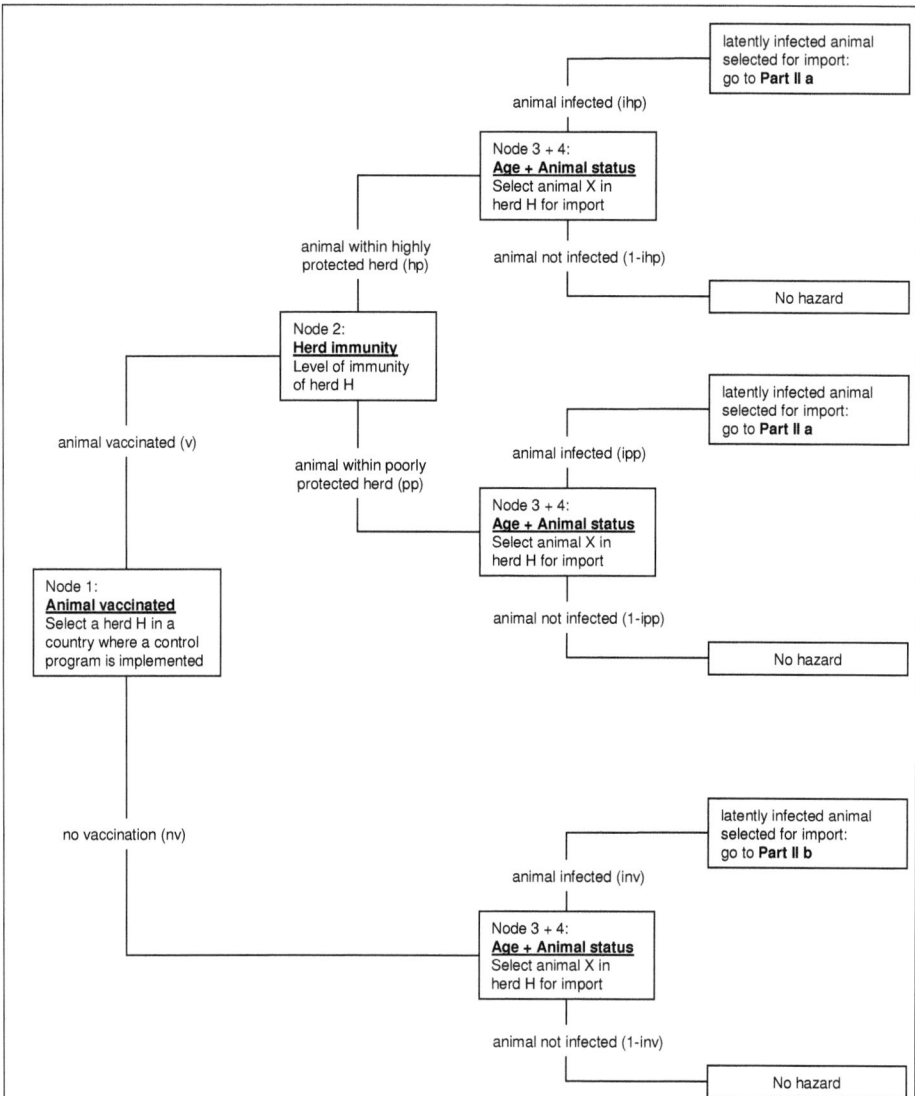

Figure 12. Release assessment for IBR, Part I: Selection of animal

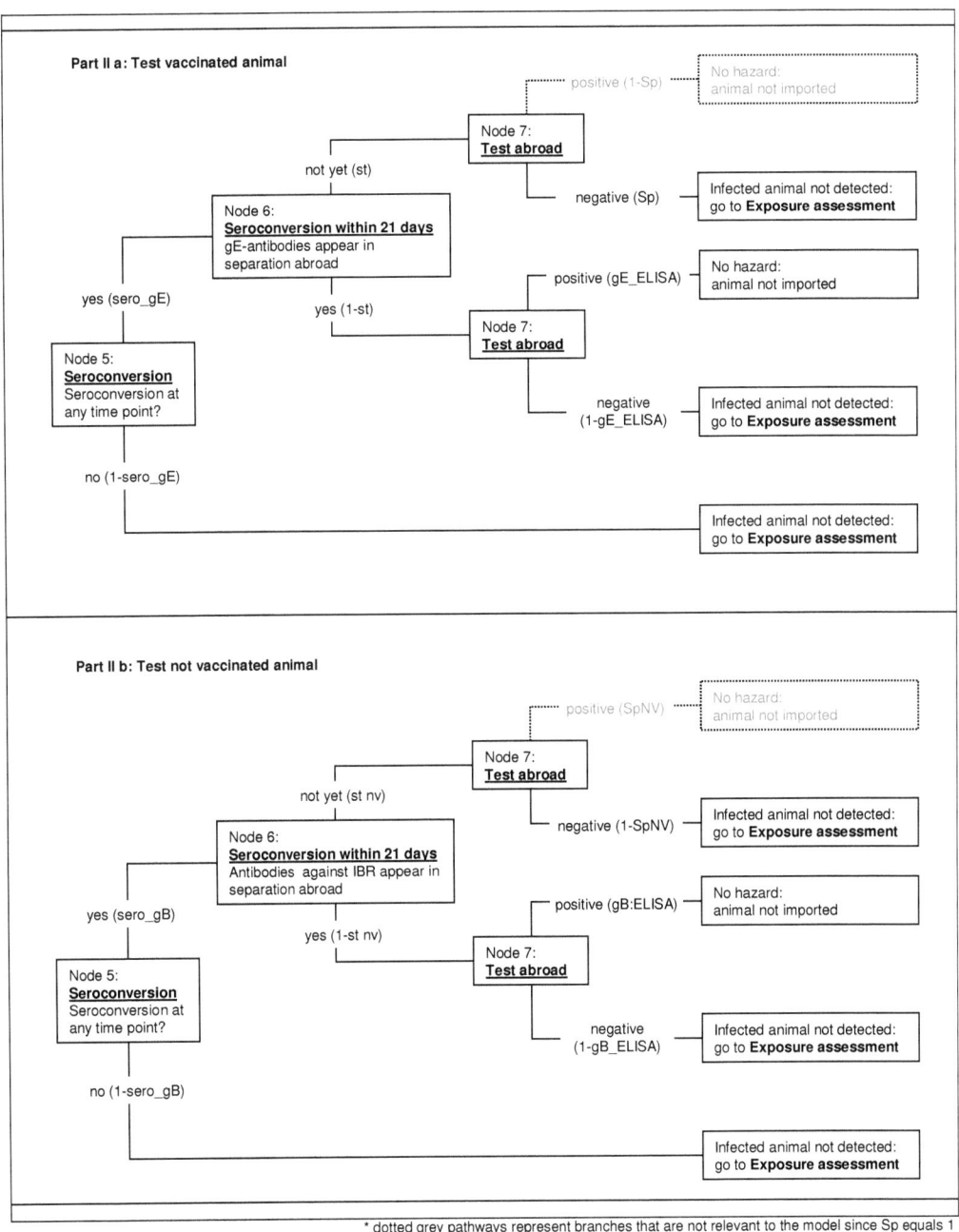

Figure 13. Release assessment for IBR, Part II: Quarantine and testing abroad

3.6.2.2. Exposure assessment

The exposure assessment describes the steps from arrival in Switzerland until introduction into domestic herd and subsequent infection of a domestic cattle. Therefore, it provides the probability, that a domestic cattle would get infected if a latently infected animal was imported as shown in Figures 14 and 15. It was divided into two parts, separation in Switzerland and introduction into domestic herd.

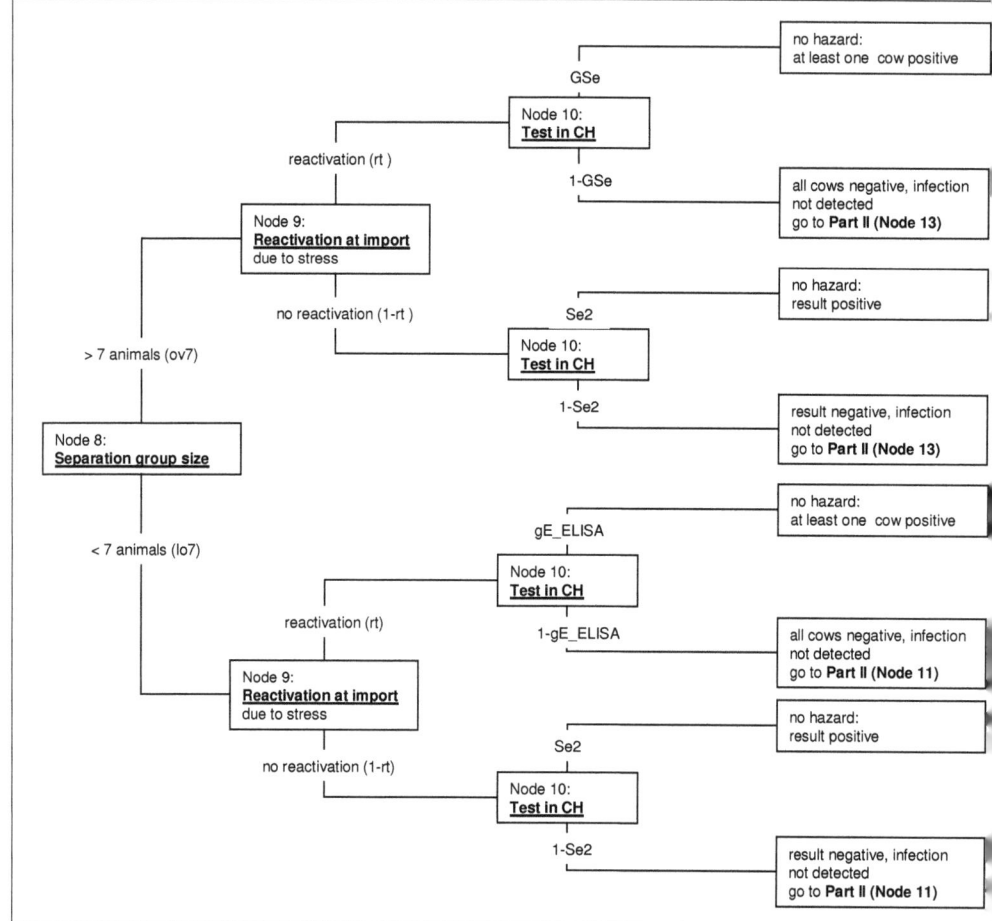

Figure 14. Exposure assessment for IBR, Part I: Separation in CH

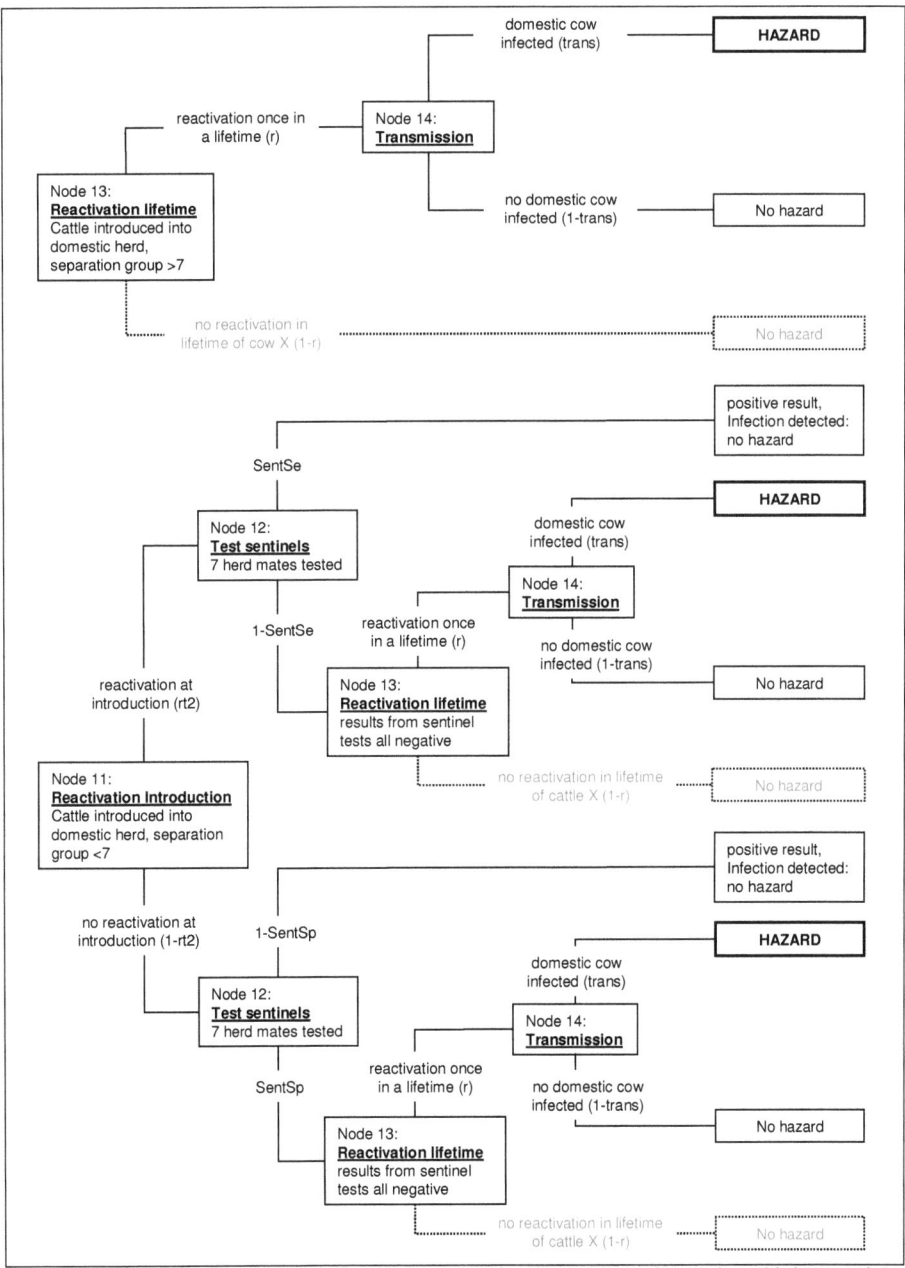

* dotted grey pathways represent branches that are not relevant to the model, since r equals 1

Figure 15. Exposure assessment for IBR, Part II; Introduction into domestic herd

3.6.3. Overview and used parameters

In Table XII, an overview of the modelled processes and a summary of the different steps within the model is given. The input parameters and abbreviations are defined in Table XIII.

Table XII. Model overview for IBR

Model IBR

Node	Name	Type	Outcome	Next Node	Data source
1	Animal vaccinated	Category risk	yes no	2 3	Input
2	Herd immunity	Category risk	highly protected poorly protected	3 3	Estimate based on literature and expert opinion
3	Age	Category risk	Q1 Q2 Q3 Q4	4 4 4 4	Data from TVD for imported cattle 2000 - 2005
4	Animal status	Infection	infected not infected	5 No hazard	Prevalence and risk for each age class derived from literature
5	Seroconversion	Category detection	yes no	6 8	Estimate based on literature and expert opinion
6	Seroconversion in 21 days	Category detection	yes not yet	7 8	Calculation based on literature and expert opinion
7	Test abroad	Detection	negative positive	8 No hazard	EFSA Opinion
8	Separation group size	Category detection	< 7 > 7	9 9	Estimate from Knopf (2004)
9	Reactivation Import	Category detection	yes no	10 10	Estimate based on literature and expert opinion
10	Test CH	Detection	negative positive	11 No hazard	EFSA Opinion and calculations for dependence and group sensitivities (sheet 'Sensitivities')
11	Reactivation Introduction	Category detection	yes no	12 12	Estimate based on literature and expert opinion
12	Test sentinels	Detection	negative positive	13 No hazard	Calculations for group sensitivity + specificity (sheet 'Sensitivities')
13	Reactivation lifetime	Category risk	yes no	14 No hazard	Estimate based on literature and expert opinion (Pert distribution with same input as for node 9)
14	Transmission	Category risk	yes no	**Hazard** No hazard	Estimate based on literature and expert opinion

Table XIII. Definitions for parameters used in the IBR model

Nr.	Node	Name	Description
1	Animal vaccinated	v	Proportion of vaccinated animals for import
		nv	Proportion of non-vaccinated animals for import
2	Herd immunity	hp	Proportion of highly protected vaccinated herds
		pp	Proportion of poorly protected vaccinated herds
3	Age	Q1	Proportion of animals < 14 months imported from 2000 to 2005
		Q2	Proportion of animals at 15 - 29 months imported from 2000 to 2005
		Q3	Proportion of animals at 30 - 48 months imported from 2000 to 2005
		Q4	Proportion of animals > 49 months imported from 2000 to 2005
4	Animal status	ihp	Probability of being infected in a vaccinated animal from highly protected herd
		ipp	Probability of being infected in a vaccinated animal from poorly protected herd
		inv	Probability of being infected in a non-vaccinated animal
		Inherdprev_hp	Prevalence within a highly protected herd
		Inherdprev_pp	Prevalence within a poorly protected herd
		Inherdprev_nv	Prevalence within a non-vaccinated herd
		HPrev	Prevalence between negative tested herds
		Inc	Incidence reported by the country of origin
		D	Time interval between two sampling rounds of the surveillance programme
		rrQ1	Relative risk for being infected of an animal within age class 1
		rrQ2	Relative risk for being infected of an animal within age class 2
		rrQ3	Relative risk for being infected of an animal within age class 3
		rrQ4	Relative risk for being infected of an animal within age class 4
		arQ1	Adjusted risk for being infected of an animal within age class 1
		arQ2	Adjusted risk for being infected of an animal within age class 2
		arQ3	Adjusted risk for being infected of an animal within age class 3
		arQ4	Adjusted risk for being infected of an animal within age class 4
		EPIhpQ1	Effective probability of being infected for a vaccinated animal from a highly protected herd within age class 1
		EPIhpQ2	Effective probability of being infected for a vaccinated animal from a highly protected herd within age class 2
		EPIhpQ3	Effective probability of being infected for a vaccinated animal from a highly protected herd within age class 3
		EPIhpQ4	Effective probability of being infected for a vaccinated animal from a highly protected herd within age class 4
		EPIppQ1	Effective probability of being infected for a vaccinated animal from a poorly protected herd within age class 1
		EPIppQ2	Effective probability of being infected for a vaccinated animal from a poorly protected herd within age class 2
		EPIppQ3	Effective probability of being infected for a vaccinated animal from a poorly protected herd within age class 3
		EPIppQ4	Effective probability of being infected for a vaccinated animal from a poorly protected herd within age class 4

		EPInvQ1	Effective probability of being infected for a non-vaccinated animal within age class 1
		EPInvQ2	Effective probability of being infected for a non-vaccinated animal within age class 2
		EPInvQ3	Effective probability of being infected for a non-vaccinated animal within age class 3
		EPInvQ4	Effective probability of being infected for a non-vaccinated animal within age class 4
5	Seroconversion	sero_gE	Proportion of vaccinated animals that seroconvert after infection
		sero_gB	Proportion of non-vaccinated animals that seroconvert after infection
6	Seroconversion in 21 days	conv_gE	Days until seroconversion for gE-antibodies in vaccinated animals
		conv_gB	Days until seroconversion for gB-antibodies in non-vaccinated animals
		ageQ1	Age of an animal from age class 1
		ageQ2	Age of an animal from age class 2
		ageQ3	Age of an animal from age class 3
		ageQ4	Age of an animal from age class 4
		stQ1	Probability of testing a vaccinated animal from age class 1 before seroconversion
		stQ2	Probability of testing a vaccinated animal from age class 2 before seroconversion
		stQ3	Probability of testing a vaccinated animal from age class 3 before seroconversion
		stQ4	Probability of testing a vaccinated animal from age class 4 before seroconversion
		stQ1nv	Probability of testing a non-vaccinated animal from age class 1 before seroconversion
		stQ2nv	Probability of testing a non-vaccinated animal from age class 2 before seroconversion
		stQ3nv	Probability of testing a non-vaccinated animal from age class 3 before seroconversion
		stQ4nv	Probability of testing a non-vaccinated animal from age class 4 before seroconversion
7	Test abroad	gE_ELISA	Sensitivity of the gE-ELISA for vaccinated animals
		gB_ELISA	Sensitivity of the gB-ELISA for non-vaccinated animals
8	Separation group size	>7	Proportion of animals separated in CH in groups with less than 7 animals
		<7	Proportion of animals separated in CH in groups 7 or more animals
9	Reactivation import	rt	Probability of reactivation of latent infection in a vaccinated animal through import stress
		rtNV	Probability of reactivation of latent infection in a non-vaccinated animal through import stress
10	Test CH	GSe_lo7	Group level sensitivity for non-vaccinated group mates of a vaccinated infected animal, while the animal itself has not seroconverted (in separation groups with less than 7 animals)
		GSe_lo7NV	Group level sensitivity for non-vaccinated group mates of a non-vaccinated infected animal, while the animal itself has not seroconverted (in separation groups with less than 7 animals)

		GSe_lo7VV	Group level sensitivity for vaccinated group mates of a vaccinated infected animal, while the animal itself has not seroconverted (in separation groups with less than 7 animals)
		GSe_ov7	Group level sensitivity for non-vaccinated group mates of a vaccinated infected animal, while the animal itself has not seroconverted (in separation groups with 7 or more animals)
		GSe_ov7NV	Group level sensitivity for non-vaccinated group mates of a non-vaccinated infected animal, while the animal itself has not seroconverted (in separation groups with 7 or more animals)
		GSe_ov7VV	Group level sensitivity for vaccinated group mates of a vaccinated infected animal, while the animal itself has not seroconverted (in separation groups with 7 or more animals)
		GSe2_lo7	Group level sensitivity for vaccinated animals in separation groups with less than 7 animals (including group mates and animal X)
		GSe2_lo7NV	Group level sensitivity for non-vaccinated animals in separation groups with less than 7 animals (including group mates and animal X)
		GSe2_lo7VV	Group level sensitivity for groups where all animals are vaccinated with less than 7 animals (including group mates and animal)
		GSe2_ov7	Group level sensitivity for vaccinated animals in separation groups with 7 or more animals (including group mates and animal X)
		GSe2_ov7NV	Group level sensitivity for non-vaccinated animals in separation groups with 7 or more animals (including group mates and animal X)
		GSe2_ov7VV	Group level sensitivity for groups where all animals are vaccinated with 7 or more animals (including group mates and animal)
		lo7size	Separation group size for group with less than 7 animals
		Se2	Single animal sensitivity of test in Switzerland for vaccinated animals, assuming dependance between tests
		Se2NV	Single animal sensitivity of test in Switzerland for non-vaccinated animals, assuming dependance between tests
		SeBom	Single animal sensitivity of indirect ELISA for non-vaccinated animals
11	Reactivation introduction	rt2	Probability of reactivation of latent infection in a vaccinated animal through introduction into new herd (equal to rt)
		rt2NV	Probability of reactivation of latent infection in a non-vaccinated animal through introduction into new herd (equal to rtNV)
12	Test sentinels	SentSe	Sensitivity of testing of the sentinel animals if imported animal was vaccinated
		SentSeNV	Sensitivity of testing of the sentinel animals if imported animal was non-vaccinated
		SentSp_Bom	Specificity of sentinella-test of seven new herd mates with Checkit® Trachitest serum-confirmation test (Bommeli)
		SentSp_gB	Specificity of sentinella-test of seven new herd mates with gB_ELISA
13	Reactivation lifetime	r	Probability of reactivation of latent infection at any time in the life of the animal
14 / 10 / 12	Transmission / Test CH / Test sentinels	trans	Probability of virus transmission from a vaccinated animal after reactivation of latent infection to its herd mate
		transNV	Probability of virus transmission from a non-vaccinated animal after reactivation of latent infection to its herd mate
		transVV	Probability of virus transmission from a vaccinated animal after reactivation of latent infection to its vaccinated herd mate

3.6.4. Inputs and calculations for the IBR model

The described model represents the import of one single cattle from the example region Saxony-Anhalt. Saxony-Anhalt was chosen because there, IBR is still present and an eradication programme approved by the EU Commission using marker-vaccination was in operation. Therefore, reports with data on disease occurrence were available.

3.6.4.1. Node 1: Animal vaccinated (Input value)

The proportion of animals that were vaccinated (**v**) was fixed at 1 to model import of vaccinated animals. The probability for an imported animal of not being vaccinated (**nv**) is **nv = 1 - v**. For comparison, **v** and **nv** can both be fixed at 1 to compare the results, i.e. run two models, one for vaccinated and one for non-vaccinated cattle.

3.6.4.2. Node 2: Herd immunity (Input value)

We estimated the proportion of herds that were likely to reach a high herd level immunity (**hp**) through vaccination and therefore would only have minor outbreaks if the virus was introduced. In contrast, in poorly protected herds (**pp**) major outbreaks would still occur, as immunity of the majority of cattle was not sufficient to prevent infection and spread. This would lead to high inherd prevalences (de Jong and Diekmann 1992).

Bosch and co-workers (Bosch, de Jong et al. 1997; Bosch, Kaashoek et al. 1997) estimated in a field experiment R_0 in not-vaccinated dairy herds at 5.6 and in cattle vaccinated with an inactivated vaccine at 2.7. Under experimental conditions, R_0 for cattle vaccinated with a live vaccine was 0.9. Vonk Noordegraaf et. al (1998) suggested to assume $R_0 = 1.5$ for live vaccines to prevent overestimation of vaccine efficacy when used in the field. On the other hand, Bosch et al. (1997) also found inactivated marker vaccines to be more efficient in reducing field BoHV-1 excretion after reactivation than live marker vaccines. Under particular assumptions, only the fraction $(1-1/R_0)$ will lead to a major outbreak (Graat, de Jong et al. 2001; De Koeijer, Diekmann et al. 1998; de Jong and Diekmann 1992; Metz 1978).

With the suggestions above for R_0, this formula lead to 62% (=1-1/2.7) of herds vaccinated with inactivated vaccine and 33% (=1-1/1.5) of those vaccinated with live vaccine having major outbreaks and were therefore poorly protected. This assumption was supported by the experts.

We used a UNIFORM DISTRIBUTION for the probability of a vaccinated herd being poorly protected (**pp**):

Minimum 33%
Maximum 62%

(where **hp = 1 - pp**)

3.6.4.3. Node 3: Age (Input value from data set)

Age is a risk factor for infection. As animals remain life-long carriers of the virus, older cattle are more likely to be infected since they have been at risk for a longer time period.

From the animal movement database TVD we obtained data of the age in months of 3011 cattle imported into Switzerland from 2000 until 2005. This data is shown in Figure 16. We grouped them into four age classes with different risks of infection following Boelaert et. al. (2005).

Data from 2005 only was investigated, since new import regulations prohibit the import of cattle born before 1.6.2001 due to BSE prevention reasons. There were no older cattle imported in 2005. But comparing the data from 2000 until 2004, there seems to be an interest in importing cattle over 4 years of age and the model was aimed to represent a hypothetical future scenario where import of older cattle would be possible again. That was the reason for using data which did not represent the current import situation.

Definition of age classes and proportions of imported animals in each class:

Q1	< 14 months	17%
Q2	15 - 29 months	62%
Q3	30 - 48 months	14%
Q4	> 49 months	8%

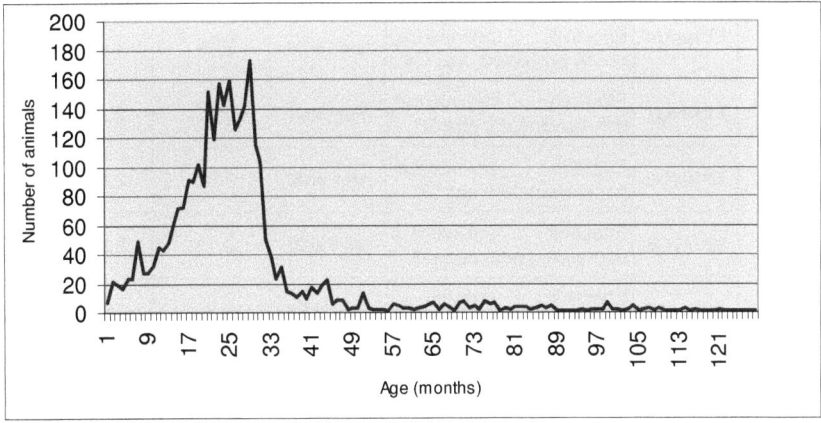

Figure 16. Age of 3011 cattle imported into Switzerland from 2000 - 2005

3.6.4.4. Node 4: Animal status (Calculation)

For each branch there was an effective probability of infection calculated to account for different risks of infection in age classes.

Effective probabilities of infection (Calculation for node 4)

To get the effective probability of infection (**EPIhpQ1; EPIhpQ2; EPIhpQ3; EPIhpQ4; EPIppQ1; EPIppQ2, EPIppQ3; EPIppQ4; EPInvQ1; EPInvQ2; EPInvQ3; EPInvQ4**) for an animal from a highly protected, poorly protected, or non-vaccinated herd within a certain age class we multiplied its probability of infection with the correspondent adjusted risk for the respective age class. The obtained values are listed in Table XIV.

$$EPI = P(infected) * adjusted\ risk\ of\ infection$$

Table XIV. Probability of infection of the animal: Effective probability of infection

Name	Definition	Formula	5th percentile	median	95th percentile
EPIhpQ1	Effective prevalence: highly protected, age Q1	*ihp * arQ1*	0.1%	0.5%	1.0%
EPIhpQ2	Effective prevalence: highly protected, age Q2	*ihp * arQ2*	0.2%	0.6%	1.2%
EPIhpQ3	Effective prevalence: highly protected, age Q3	*ihp * arQ3*	0.2%	0.8%	1.6%
EPIhpQ4	Effective prevalence: highly protected, age Q4	*ihp * arQ4*	0.3%	1.1%	2.1%

EPIppQ1	Effective prevalence: poorly protected, age Q1	ipp * arQ1	1.2%	2.2%	3.6%
EPIppQ2	Effective prevalence: poorly protected, age Q2	ipp * arQ2	1.6%	2.8%	4.3%
EPIppQ3	Effective prevalence: poorly protected, age Q3	ipp * arQ3	2.1%	3.8%	6.1%
EPIppQ4	Effective prevalence: poorly protected, age Q4	ipp * arQ4	2.7%	4.9%	7.8%
EPInvQ1	Effective prevalence: non-vaccinated, age Q1	inv * arQ1	1.2%	2.2%	3.7%
EPInvQ2	Effective prevalence: non-vaccinated, age Q2	inv * arQ2	1.5%	2.8%	4.3%
EPInvQ3	Effective prevalence: non-vaccinated, age Q3	inv * arQ3	2.1%	3.8%	6.2%
EPInvQ4	Effective prevalence: non-vaccinated, age Q4	inv * arQ4	2.7%	4.9%	7.9%

Probability of infection (Calculation for node 4)

Probability of infection of the imported animal (**ihp; ipp; inv**) was derived from herd prevalence (**HPrev**) and the respective inherd prevalence for highly protected (**Inherdprev_hp**), poorly protected (**Inherdprev_pp**) and non-vaccinated herds (**Inherdprev_nv**) as follows. The obtained values are shown in Table XV.

P(animal infected) = HPrev * Inherdprev

Table XV. Probability of infection of the animal: Values calculated for herd type

Name	Definition	Formula	5th percentile	median	95th percentile
ihp	Animal status / prevalence: from highly protected herd	HPrev * Inherdprev_hp	0.19%	0.65%	1.24%
ipp	Animal status / prevalence: from poorly protected herd	HPrev * Inherdprev_pp	1.70%	2.99%	4.65%
inv	Animal status / prevalence: non-vaccinated herd	HPrev * Inherdprev_nv	1.69%	3.00%	4.63%

Inherd prevalences (Input value for node 4)

We estimated the prevalence within an infected herd for
- highly protected herds where only minor outbreaks occur (**Inherdprev_hp**)
- poorly protected herds where major outbreaks are very likely (**Inherdprev_pp**)
- non-vaccinated herds (**Inherdprev_nv**)

Transmission probability and mean duration of infectivity in vaccinated animals varies strongly with the level of herd protection (de Jong, 1995; de Jong and Diekmann, 1992). Therefore, we suggested dealing with inherd prevalence as dependent from immunity on herd level. This assumption was supported by literature data, showing that within infected herds the inherd prevalence was either very low or rather high. Defining two types of herds helped to overcome the problem of representing inherd prevalence as a distribution with two peaks by using two one-peak distributions.

To get a biologically plausible overall distribution for inherd prevalence, we allowed for an overlap of the two distributions by implementing the estimated maximal value for highly protected herds as the minimum value for poorly protected herds and vice versa.

A mean inherd prevalence of 20% was reported in the Maastrich papers (Anonymous, 1997). The model of Vonk Noordegraaf et. al. (1998) calculated national prevalence of gE-positive cattle in equilibrium at 23% with average inherd prevalence in vaccinated herds at 12% but inherd prevalence varied greatly between different herd types (Bosch et al., 1998; Bosch et al., 1997). After discussion with the expert group we assumed the following values: For highly protected herds inherd prevalences from 0.1 % to 20% with a most likely value of 10% and for poorly protected herds, a most likely value of 50% within a range between 30% and 100%. This lead to the following Pert distributions, implementing the estimated values as suggested above:

inherd prevalence for highly protected herd (**Inherdprev_hp**)
    Minimum 0.1%
    Most likely 10%
    Maximum 30%

inherd prevalence for poorly protected herd (**Inherdprev_pp**)
    Minimum 20%
    Most likely 50%
    Maximum 100%

For non-vaccinated herds (**Inherdprev_nv**) our experts expected the same inherd prevalence once the herd was infected as for poorly protected herds.

Herd prevalence (Calculation for node 4)

Herd level prevalence (**HPrev**) was calculated from apparent herd level incidence rate (**Inc**) and the duration until next testing (**D**) with the following formula (Thrusfield, 2005). Incidence rate was used since only certified BoHV-1 free herds were qualified for export to Switzerland. Therefore, not prevalence of infected herds in the country but number of newly infected herds between two sampling rounds was relevant to the model. This is consistent with the method suggested by the EFSA report on BoHV-1 free animals and establishments (Anonymous, 2005b).

$$\text{HPrev} = \text{Inc} * D$$

Herd incidence (Input value for node 4)

Apparent incidence rate (**Inc**) was modelled as a Gamma distribution. Data from our example region, Saxony-Anhalt, was 123 new positive within 2205 formerly negative herds in 2004 (Denzin and Ewert, 2005). Mean incidence was estimated at 5.7%. Incidence rate is by definition the proportion of newly infected herds to total herd years at risk (Thrusfield, 2005). Herd years at risk were calculated as follows:

((2392 herds - 187 infected at beginning of year)+(2392 herds - 310 infected at end of year) / 2

Saxony-Anhalt was chosen as an example region because an official eradication programme was implemented and there were vaccinated as well as non-vaccinated herds in the area.

Surveillance programme in the country (Input value for node 4)

The time between two sampling rounds in years (**D**) to calculate herd prevalence from herd incidence was derived from the regulations for the surveillance programme of the country. In Saxony-Anhalt herds were sampled once a year to maintain their status (Denzin and Ewert, 2005).

Relative risk of infection (Input value for node 4)

The risk of being infected is relative to the age of the animal; therefore we defined a relative risk of being infected for animals within specified age classes.

To calculate the relative risk of infection, we estimated prevalences for each age class. Boelaert reported 24% (CI 18-30), 29% (CI 22-36), 40% (CI 33-48), and 51% (CI 44-59) for the age classes **Q1, Q2, Q3**, and **Q4** respectively (Boelaert, Speybroeck et al. 2005). This data refers to the Belgian cattle population and might not be representative for other countries relating to numbers. But we were only using the ratio between prevalences in the different age classes and we assumed comparable relations between age and prevalence for other European countries.

We estimated prevalences as Beta distributions, using the RiskBetaGeneralAlt-function of @RISK that allows designing a Beta distribution by defining confidence interval and minimum and maximum value. To calculate relative risk per age class as a ratio of estimated prevalences we had to assure that estimated prevalence was not smaller than the prevalence of the next younger age class. This problem was solved by using an Excel If-function. The used distributions and the If-function are shown in Table XVI.

Table XVI. Relative risks of infection for different age classes

	Beta distribution for prevalence				Control	
	2.5%	97.5%	min	max	@RISK distribution: RiskBetaGeneralAlt	If	then
Q1	0.18	0.30	0	1	(0.025;0.18;0.975;0.30;"min";0;"max";1)	no If-function	
Q2	0.22	0.36	0	1	(0.025;0.22;0.975;0.36;"min";0;"max";1)	Q2 < Q1	= Q1
Q3	0.33	0.48	0	1	(0.025;0.33;0.975;0.48;"min";0;"max";1)	Q3 < Q2	= Q2
Q4	0.44	0.55	0	1	(0.025;0.44;0.975;0.55;"min";0;"max";1)	Q4 < Q3	= Q3

Per definition, relative risks are estimated from data or expert opinion and specified relative to the lowest risk branch (= relative risk of lowest branch is 1). We fixed the relative risk of being infected as 1 for **Q1**. The corresponding risk factors for the other age classes were then calculated as a proportion to **rrQ1** by dividing the estimated prevalence for each age class by the prevalence estimated for **Q1**.

rrQ2 = estimated prevalence in Q2 divided by estimated prevalence in Q1

rrQ3 = estimated prevalence in Q3 divided by estimated prevalence in Q1

rrQ4 = estimated prevalence in Q4 divided by estimated prevalence in Q1

Adjusted risk of infection (Calculation for node 4)

Relative risks, specified relative to the lowest risk branch, had to be adjusted to ensure that the weighted average risk for the reference population was 1 (Thrusfield, 2005). In our case, this meant

$$arQ1 * Q1 + arQ2 * Q2 + arQ3 * Q3 + arQ4 * Q4 = 1$$

and **adjusted risk** = relative risk * adjusted risk for lowest risk branch

The inputs for the relative risk (**rrQ1; rrQ2; rrQ3; rrQ4**) for each age class were explained above. To calculate the adjusted risk for the respective age class (**arQ1; arQ2; arQ3; arQ4**), based on the proportion of animal present within each class, we used the following formulas.

$$arQ1 = 1 / (Q1 + rrQ2 * Q2 + rrQ3 * Q3 + rrQ4 * Q4)$$

$$arQ2 = rrQ2 * arQ1 \text{ and so on...}$$

3.6.4.5. Node 5: Seroconversion (Input value)

There are cases reported in literature where infected animals did not seroconvert at all. These seronegative carriers were mostly due to infections when maternal antibodies were still present at high level. It is also most likely that there is biological variance between individuals and their immunological response.

Hage et al. (1996) concluded from their experiments that cattle can be seronegative against gB and gE but still carry BoHV-1 in a latent form and suggested that there exist completely BoHV-1 seronegative animals that are latently infected. Five of the six investigated seronegative heifers that had been vaccinated in presence of maternal antibodies shed virus after dexamethasone treatment at the age of tree years. Toussaint et al. (2004) immunised twenty-four calves four times before challenge with small doses of BoHV-1. The five calves that shed virus after the challenge showed no delay in seroconversion compared to non-vaccinated controls. But nineteen calves, where strong immunity prevented detectable virus replication and gE-seroconversion, stayed negative. Using PCR, BoHV-1 could be detected in the trigeminal ganglia of seven of the gE-seronegative, challenge-infected calves indicating that they were seronegative carriers (58% of at least twelve latently infected calves).

On the other hand, Schynts et. al. (2001) found four of six calves possessing high levels of maternal antibodies from vaccinated cows positive against gE five weeks after low dose infection. But even with repeated dexamethasone treatment, virus could not be reactivated in the two gE-negative calves, and was not detected in the trigeminal ganglion. Furthermore, the animals also turned negative in the gB-ELISA once maternal antibodies faded out. This suggests, that the two calves were really uninfected.

The experts agreed on the following probabilities based on literature. We assumed the same values for non-vaccinated animals as the effects of maternal antibodies were thought to be similar for calves from vaccinated and non-vaccinated cows.

We are using a PERT DISTRIBUTION for probability of seroconversion (**sero_gE; sero_gB**)

> minimum 95%
> most likely 100%
> maximum 100%

3.6.4.6. Node 6: Seroconversion in 21 days (Calculation)

The probability of seroconversion in an infected animal at time of testing abroad (**stQ1; stQ2; stQ3; stQ4; stQ1nv; stQ2nv; stQ3nv; stQ4nv**) was calculated. Cattle had to be separated for thirty days and tested for BoHV-1 at earliest after twenty-one days in separation in the country of origin. Animals that seroconverted before twenty-one days would therefore be detected anyway and **sero_gE** equaled 1. To account for this we used an If-function in excel. For animals that seroconverted more than twenty-one days after infection, we calculated the risk that it had been infected exactly within the last days before separation as follows:

$$st = 1 - ((conv\_gE - 21) / age)$$

This formula was based on the assumption of a daily risk of infection for each day in the life of a cattle which can be calculated as 1 divided by the age in days. This suggests that the risk of infection is constant for each day, which is certainly untrue. We justified this simplification with the assumption that the higher susceptibility in younger animals (especially before vaccination) and the augmented risk due to stress and handling in older animals equal each other.

Using this simplification for the daily risk of infection allowed us to multiply the daily risk by the estimated days until seroconversion minus the twenty-one days until sampling to calculate the probability of testing an animal exactly within these critical days before seroconversion and therefore missing the infection.

The age of the animal was derived as a cumulative distribution from the data set obtained from TVD. Data was divided according to the defined age classes, cumulative probabilities calculated within each class and a cumulative distribution derived as an estimate for age of the animal. The outcome was converted from months into days and rounded to full days (**ageQ1, ageQ2, ageQ3, ageQ4**). For age class **Q1** we had to adjust for cases where age was smaller than time until seroconversion because an animal could not get infected before birth and in those cases probability for seroconversion before testing was zero.

stQ1 (age>conv_gE;conv_gE>21) = 1 - ((conf_gE - 21) / ageQ1)
stQ2 (conv_gE>21) = 1 - ((conf_gE - 21) / ageQ2) and so on...

stQ1nv (age>conv_gB;conv_gE>21) = 1 - ((conf_gB - 21) / ageQ1)
stQ2nv (conv_gB>21) = 1 - ((conf_gB - 21) / ageQ2) and so on...

Days until seroconversion (Input value for node 6)

For animals that do seroconvert, the number of days until detectable seroconversion after infection (**conv_gE; conv_gB**) was estimated as a Pert distribution. In experiments, most animals were tested positive for gE-antibodies two weeks after infection, latest reported after thirty-five days (Beer et al., 2003; Schynts et al., 2001). Seroconversion against gE in vaccinated animals always took a couple of days more than seroconversion in non-vaccinated animals. For non-vaccinated animals, a maximum of ten days was reported by Beer et. al. (2003). Kramps et al. (2004) described one case that was still negative on day eighteen after infection but positive after 1120 days. The other twenty-three infected animals had all turned positive by day eleven. As we lacked of knowledge on the exact time of seroconversion of this one particular cattle, we assumed the same maximum for gB-antibodies as reported for gE.

Antibodies against gB were first detected on day eight and nine, respectively (Beer et al., 2003; Kramps et al., 2004). For gE-antibodies Beer et al. (2003) reported a minimum of fourteen days, which is congruent with Kaashoek et. al. (1996). Unfortunately, in most gE-ELISA experiments, testing was only done once a week and therefore negative animals on day seven that where positive on day fourteen must have seroconverted anytime between eight and thirteen days.

We used a PERT DISTRIBUTION for time until seroconversion after infection for

vaccinated cattle: gE-antibodies (**conv_gE**)
        minimum 9 days
        most likely 14 days
        maximum 35 days

and for non-vaccinated cattle: gB-antibodies (**conv_gB**)
minimum 8 days
most likely 9 days
maximum 35 days

3.6.4.7. Node 7: Test abroad (Input value)

Sensitivity of gE-ELISA (Input value for node 7: vaccinated animals)

The marker diagnostic kits to detect antibodies against gE have been evaluated in an European trial and the EFSA-Opinion on BoHV-1 free establishments referred to these results (Kramps et al., 2004, Anonymous, 2005b).

We used a PERT DISTRIBUTION for sensitivity of gE-blocking-ELISA (**gE_ELISA**) with
minimum 59%
most likely 72%
maximum 85%

Sensitivity of gB-ELISA (Input value for node 7: non-vaccinated animals)

The EFSA-Opinion on BoHV-1 free establishments recommended the use of gB-ELISAs as the most sensitive screening test with better performance than other ELISAs detecting more or different antibodies (Anonymous, 2005b). Performance was also referred to Kramps et al. (2004).

We used a PERT DISTRIBUTION for sensitivity of gB-blocking-ELISA (**gB_ELISA**) with
minimum 69%
most likely 96%
maximum 100%

Specificity (Input value for node 7)

Specificity was seen as 100% for the tests applied to the animal abroad and after separation in Switzerland, because positive test results would be further investigated with confirmatory tests. Only for the sentinel test in the destined Swiss herd specificity was taken into account, since a positive result in a sentinel animal, even if false positive, would lead to retesting of the imported animal and further investigation.

3.6.4.8. Node 8: Separation group size (Input value)

After import, cattle from not officially IBR-free countries were separated for three weeks and afterwards tested serologically. Specifications for proceeding animals from separation groups with seven or more animals (**ov7**) and from separation groups with less than seven animals (**lo7**) were different. In larger separation groups, group sensitivity enlarged the probability to detect the infection. In small groups, probability of detection was increased by testing the animal's new herd mates in its destination establishment after another three weeks as sentinel animals. As we, in fact, had no knowledge on separation group sizes of cattle imports we assumed 50% of the animals in groups with less and more than seven animals, respectively (Knopf et. al., 2004.

3.6.4.9. Node 9: Reactivation during import (Input value)

The probability of reactivation in a latently infected animal during import and separation (**rt**) was estimated as a Pert distribution. Transportation and crowding means stress and might provoke a reactivation in latently infected animals as seen in the case of cattle import from France in 2005. But there were not many experiments on reactivation of

BoHV-1 in latently infected vaccinated cattle and the used model (dexamethasone treatment) simulated a very high level of stress (Tanaka, 2003).

Vonk Noordegraaf et al. (1998) estimated in their model the probability of virus reactivation in a gE-positive animal upon transport, followed by transmission of the virus on the receiving farm, as 0.07. Kaashoek et. al. (1996) could reactivate latent infection in three out of four vaccinated animals (75%). Van Oirschot et al. (1996a) could provoke virus reactivation with dexamethasone in only one out of eight vaccinated calves (13%).

Our conclusion after discussion with the experts was a PERT DISTRIBUTION for the probability of reactivation in vaccinated animal at import (**rt**) with

minimum 1%
most likely 13%
maximum 75%

Non-vaccinated latently infected animals are much more likely to reactivate infection at import. We estimated a PERT DISTRIBUTION for **rtNV** with the opinion of our experts.

minimum 25%
most likely 50%
maximum 75%

3.6.4.10. Node 10: Test CH (Calculation)

Several points had to be taken into account concerning testing in Switzerland after three weeks of separation. If the latent infection was reactivated, separation group mates might be infected and therefore test sensitivity increased due to group sensitivity. On the other hand, without reactivation, the infected animal could only be identified by testing the animal itself and therefore, only single test sensitivity applied.

In the current situation, the indirect ELISA was used in Switzerland. If cattle in separation abroad had been tested with gB-ELISA as recommended by EFSA (Anonymous, 2005b), the test in Switzerland had full sensitivity because there was no dependence. Should this situation change and Switzerland would adopt the gB-ELISA too, the test applied to the infected animal would be semi-dependent because it would be the same animal but four weeks later with the same test but a different batch in a different laboratory. For vaccinated animals, gE-ELISA was used on both occasions, therefore dependence between tests had to be taken into account.

Group sensitivity for less than seven animals (Calculation for node 10)

First we calculateed the effective number of animals in the group or, more precisely, the number of group mates of an infected animal. For the groups with less than seven animals we made the same assumption as Knopf et. al. (2004): 5% are groups with only one animal, 15% with three animals and 80% contain five animals. This lead to a cumulative probability for each situation of 0.05, 0.2, and 1, respectively. We modelled the number of group mates (**lo7size**) as a cumulative distribution with a minimum of zero and a maximum of six for an import group with seven or less animals.

The model of Knopf et al. (2004) was used to calculate group sensitivity (**GSe2_lo7; GSe2_lo7NV; GSe2_lo7VV**) for each group size of herd mates in separation based on test sensitivity, transmission probabilities, and binomial distribution of infected group mates.

Since the originally infected animal was retested, too, sensitivity of that test had to be added to the calculated group sensitivity to get the sensitivity for the whole group including the latently infected animal. For the formerly not infected group mates, the full sensitivity of the ELISA applied but for the formerly false negative animal, this sampling represented a second test. Since reactivation of the infection occurred in the animal and virus was shed between the two tests, we assumed a relevant change in its immunological situation and therefore independence between testing (full sensitivity of the ELISA).

vaccinated animal, group non-vaccinated: GSe2_lo7 = 1 - (1 - gE_ELISA) * (1 - GSe_lo7)
all animals non-vaccinated: GSe2_lo7NV = 1 - (1 - gB_ELISA) * (1 - GSe_lo7NV)
all animals vaccinated: GSe2_lo7VV = 1 - (1 - gB_ELISA) * (1 - GSe_lo7VV)

Because we only used group sensitivity when reactivation of the latent infection in the originally infected animal had occurred, we could use the estimated value for virus transmission once the animal had reactivated (**trans; transNV; transVV**) for transmission probability.

In case of no seroconversion in the originally infected animal (node 5), group sensitivity for separation herd mates was still applicable after reactivation and transmission (**GSe_lo7; GSe_lo7NV; GSe_lo7VV**).

Group sensitivity for more than seven animals (Calculation)

Differences in group sensitivities get smaller, the larger the group. Therefore, group sensitivities for larger groups (**GSe2_ov7; GSe2_ov7NV; GSe2_ov7VV; GSe_ov7; GSe_ov7NV; GSe_ov7VV**) were not calculated as detailed as for small ones. We used the same model as for small groups and calculated the values for GSe for seven, ten, and thirty animals, respectively, and implemented those values in a Pert distribution as minimal, most likely, and maximal value. These were just assumptions on group size of large import groups (min. 7, ml. 10, max. 30) since there was no available data. The minimal value was first estimated and then implemented as a fixed value of 99% to overcome calculation problems in Microsoft Excel. Several If-functions were used to assure that the most likely value was equal or smaller than the maximum value.

Sensitivity of Bommeli ELISA (Input value for node 10)

In Switzerland, for IBR screening, the indirect Bommeli ELISA (Checkit® Trachitest) was still in use. Its performance was estimated following Kramps et. al. (2004) and EFSA-Opinion (Anonymous, 2005b).

We used a PERT DISTRIBUTION for sensitivity of indirect ELISA (**Se_Bom**) with
minimum 69%
most likely 87%
maximum 94%

Sensitivity of dependent test (Input value for node 10)

The animals were first tested abroad after at least twenty-one days in separation and shipped about nine days later as separation was compulsory for thirty days. In Switzerland, the animals were kept separately for another twenty-one days before retesting (Anonymous, 2005d; Anonymous, 2004a).

So the two ELISAs were only partially depending:
- The same animal but four weeks later
- Same test but different batch or same testing principle but from different producer
- Different laboratory

To calculate sensitivity of the second dependent test (**Se2; Se2NV**) it is recommended to calculate the proportion of positive results after prior false negatives (Thrusfield, 2005). Kramps et al. (2004) showed the results of different laboratories where all sera were tested twice. This approach showed complete dependence as the same sera were tested in the same lab at the same time.

For the gE-ELISAs with samples known to be positive there were forty-four pairs with at least one negative or doubtful result. In eight of those cases, the second result was positive and infection would have been detected with the second test. This would lead to sensitivity for second test of 0.18. Only thirty-seven of the tests showed at least one negative result and ten of them could have been detected, as the second result was either positive or doubtful. The proportion would therefore be 0.27.

For gB-ELISA there were seventeen pairs with at least one negative or doubtful result of which five had a positive result and would have been detected with a probability of 0.29. Only eleven of them had actually at least one negative result and six could have been recognised due to a positive or doubtful second test result. This would lead to a sensitivity of second test of 0.55.

We calculated confidence intervals for those estimates and modelled sensitivity of the second, dependent test as a Beta distribution using the RiskBetaGeneralAlt-function in @risk with 2.5% percentile, 97.5% percentile, minimum zero and as maximum the maximal value from the pert distribution estimating test sensitivity. Then we simulated the confidence interval values as uniform distributions, using the calculated values for both extremes (as explained above) as minimum and maximum. With those values we created a new Beta distribution for sensitivity of the second test, combining the two extremes using again the RiskBetaGeneralAlt-function in @risk. This was done for both, the gE_ELISA and the gB_ELISA and the obtained values are shown in Table XVII.

Sensitivity of dependent test would be needed for non-vaccinated animals, if Switzerland would conduct a gB-ELISA. Presently, the indirect Bommeli ELISA (Checkit® Trachitest) for detection of the whole antibody spectrum, which represents not only a different test but also a different testing principle (indirect ELISA vs. blocking ELISA) was used. Therefore, sampling in Switzerland after three weeks was independent and had full sensitivity of indirect ELISA. For vaccinated animals, Switzerland would use a gE-ELISA, too, and therefore we had to account for test dependence concerning vaccinated animals, that have already seroconverted before test abroad (node 6) and without reactivation of infection at import (node 9). After reactivation and virus shedding, we assumed independence between tests as the immunological situation of the animal had changed.

Table XVII. Submodel sensitivities: Values obtained for sensitivity of dependent tests

Name	Definition	Formula	5th percentile	median	95th percentile
Se2	Sensitivity of second gE-ELISA, assuming test dependence	Beta distribution from data	12.3%	23.0%	36.4%
Se2NV	Sensitivity of second gB-ELISA, assuming test dependence	Beta distribution from data	77.0%	85.6%	91.8%

3.6.4.11. Node 11: Reactivation at introduction (Input value equal to node 9)

After separation, the imported cattle was introduced into a Swiss domestic herd. This required transportation and handling for integration of the animal into its new herd and could lead to reactivation of latent infection.

The experts assessed the stress due to import as comparable to the stress at introduction into determined herd after separation in Switzerland. Therefore, for reactivation at introduction, we used the same input values as for node 9. But to account for different reactions of a single animal to the two stress situations, we modelled probability of reactivation at introduction (**rt2; rt2NV**) in a second simulation.

3.6.4.12. Node 12: Test sentinels (Calculation)

Group sensitivity for sentinel animals (Model output)

In Switzerland, after introduction of the animal into its destined herd, cattle imported in groups smaller than seven animals were retested through a sentinel approach

(Anonymous, 2004e). Instead of retesting the imported animal (third test, same animal, large test dependence leads to low sensitivity), seven of the animal's new herd mates were tested for IBR after at least four weeks but not the animal itself. Sensitivity of the sentinella-testing (*SentSe, SentSeNV*) equaled group sensitivity for seven group mates as showed for node 10 but was only relevant if reactivation of latent infection in the infected animal had occurred after introduction into its new herd (**rt2; rt2NV**). The values obtained for group sensitivity of seven herd mates are shown in Table XVIII.

Group specificity for sentinel animals (Calculation from input value)

Only for the sentinel test in the destined Swiss herd specificity was taken into account, since a positive result, even if false positive, would lead to retesting of the imported animal and further investigation.

To calculate group specificity for sentinel test, specificity was estimated following Kramps et al. (2004) and EFSA-Opinion (Anonymous, 2005b).

We used a PERT DISTRIBUTION for specificity of indirect ELISA (**Sp_Bom**) with

minimum 88%

most likely 99%

maximum 100%

For the gB-ELISA (**SentSp_gB**), Kramps reported the same specificity values as for the indirect ELISA.

Then, group specificity for sentinel test of 7 non-vaccinated Swiss herd mates, was calculated for use of Bommeli ELISA (SentSp_Bom) or gB-ELISA (SentSp_gB):

SentSp_Bom = (specificity Bommeli)^7

SentSp_gB = (specificity gB-ELISA)^7

Table XVIII. Test sentinels: Expected value for sensitivity and specificity

Name	Definition	Formula	5th percentile	median	95th percentile
SentSe	Sensitivity of testing seven sentinel animals after reactivation at introduction in infected animal	*model Knopf: 7 herd mates*	99.98%	99.9999%	100%
SentSp	Specificity of testing seven sentinel animals (if infected animal did not reactivate)	*(specificity)* ^{7}	63.24%	85.10%	97.83%

3.6.4.13. Node 13: Reactivation lifetime (Input value)

The probability of reactivation in a latently infected animal at any point in the life of a breeding or dairy cattle (**r**) was estimated by experts at 100% (Ackermann, M., Swiss reference laboratory for IBR, personal communication). We assumed for the lifetime of a cattle that there would always be at least once a stress factor strong enough to reactivate infection. Furthermore, in vaccinated animals the vaccination would no longer be boosted and immunity would probably fade out. Stress factors are, for example, parturition, crowding, transport, diseases, medical treatment and handling. On the other hand, the animal might died due to any reason and therefore did not reactivate infection within lifetime. To account for those cases and to get a biologically plausible input in absence of reliable data, we used a Uniform distribution with

Minimum 95%

Maximum 100%

3.6.4.14. Node 14: Transmission (Input value)

The probability of virus transmission to a naïve herd mate once the infection was reactivated (**trans**) was estimated as a Pert distribution. This was difficult because common experimental design involved either vaccinated or non-vaccinated cattle. Mixture of both was not part of any eradication programme specially not because the goal of vaccination was to reach a high protection on herd level rather than on single animal level. R_0 for non-vaccinated animals was estimated at 5.6 (Bosch et al., 1997), so if once one domestic animal was infected a major outbreak among our naïve population would be most likely. Hage et al. (1996) estimated R_0 as 7 in their population dynamics of BoHV-1 trial. Bosch et al. (1997) found in their experiments with different vaccines R_0 values from 0.9 for live vaccines up to 2.6 for inactivated vaccines. Vonk Noordegraaf et al. (1998) used a value of 1.5 for herds vaccinated with live vaccines in their model because in the field animals might get infected before they are effectively immunised. As mentioned above, they also estimated the probability of a latently infected, vaccinated cattle to reactivate and transmit the virus to another herd mate at 0.07. Within the present model this value would represent **rt** multiplied by **trans**. Using this value as a minimum because it referred to transmission from vaccinated to vaccinated animal we calculated 0.54 for **trans** (using the most likely value o 0.13 for **rt**). Obviously, transmission to naive contact animals is much more likely and based on the high R_0 values for non-vaccinated animals we assumed a most likely probability for transmission of 100%.

Probability of transmission of virus from vaccinated to non-vaccinated cattle (**trans**) was estimated as PERT DISTRIBUTION with

> minimum 54%
> most likely 100%
> maximum 100%

Based on the high values for R_0 for non-vaccinated animals and expert opinion we fixed **transNV** at 100%.

Transmission probability from vaccinated to vaccinated animal (**transVV**) was estimated, too, to be able to adjust the model for a whole group of vaccinated animals imported. As a first step, the model represented the situation of importing only one vaccinated cattle within an import group of non-vaccinated animals. This was reasonable, because animals from different herds are often gathered at one collecting establishment for separation before shipping and, mainly in France, heterogenous herds with vaccinated and non-vaccinated individuals exist (Anonymous, 2005c). In the following, the scenario of importing a whole group of vaccinated animals was simulated too.

3.7. SENSITIVITY ANALYSIS

The impact of variables on the outcome for both models was analysed using tornado charts based on calculated regression coefficients. Tornado charts provide a pictorial representation to illustrate sensitivity analysis of the models. The charts show to what degree individual variables influence the model output. The bar length represents the degree of association. The larger it is, the more is the respective input variable affecting the output (Vose, 2003). Positive and negative associations are indicated by the direction of the bar. Positive associated variables increase the model output while negative associated ones decrease it, when the variable itself becomes larger.

Chapter 4   Results

An important output of this project were the developed models described in Chapter 3. In this section, we present the output values derived from these models. All designations used for the variables in the tables and charts are defined in Tables 5 and 13.

4.1.   MODEL OUTPUT

4.1.1.   Aujeszky's disease

After one simulation with 10^6 iterations and input values as presented in chapter 3.5, we obtained the following outputs for the probability of introducing AD through the import of one pig. Medians as well as 5th and 95th percentiles are shown.

Marker-vaccinated pig 4.93×10^{-4} (5.83×10^{-5} - 1.60×10^{-3})

Non-vaccinated pig 4.73×10^{-7} (4.92×10^{-8} - 1.88×10^{-6})

This means that if one vaccinated pig is imported, on average one can be 99.95% confident that it would not introduce AD into Switzerland. In case of repeated imports, an undesired outcome would occur in roughly 5 out of 10,000 cases. For non-vaccinated animals, the mean value was 99.9999%.

The results indicate a 1000-fold lower probability for non-vaccinated animals. Distributions for the output values are shown in Figures 18, 19 and 20 as ascending cumulative frequency plots. They show the probability of the output being less than or equal to the x-axis value (Vose, 2003). In Figure 17 the values are presented graphically for comparison.

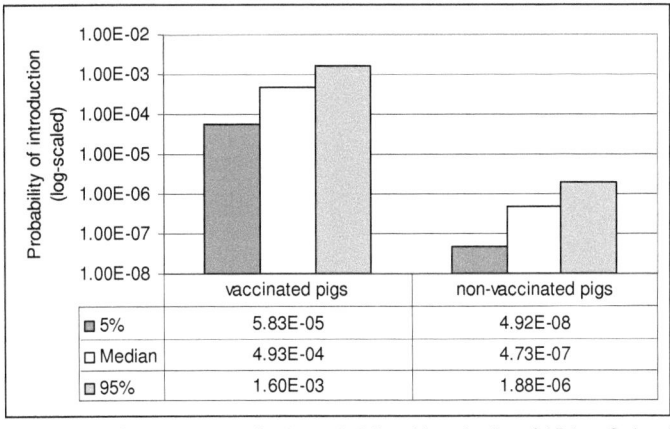

Figure 17. Obtained values for the probability of introduction of AD into Switzerland by one single imported pig

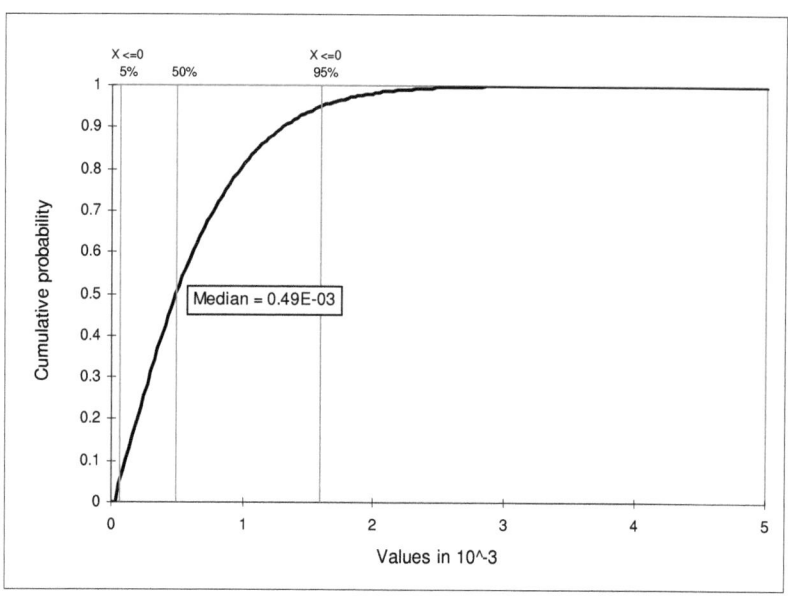

Figure 18. Cumulative distribution of the probability of AD introduction in a vaccinated pig

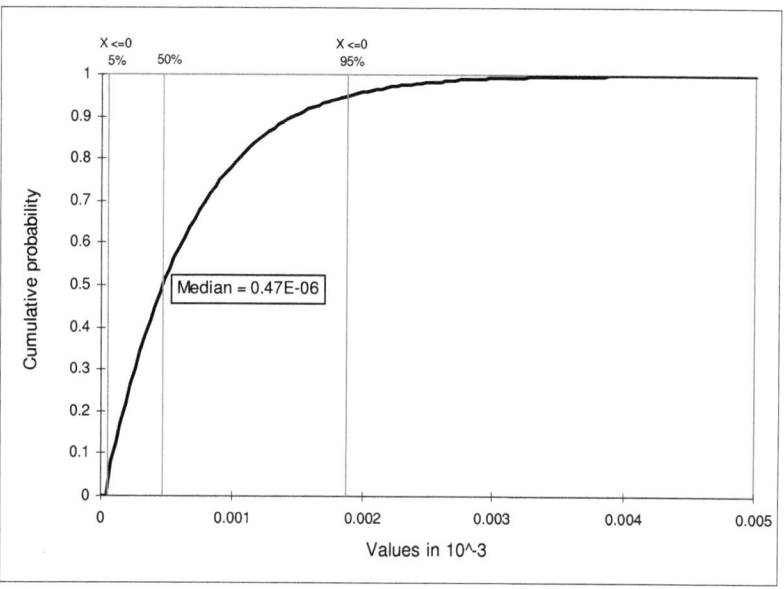

Figure 19. Cumulative distribution of the probability of AD introduction in a non-vaccinated pig

4.1.2. Infectious bovine rhinotracheitis

After one simulation with 10^6 iterations and input values as presented in Chapter 3, we obtained the following outputs for the probability of introducing IBR through the import of one cattle. Mean values as well as 5th and 95th percentiles are shown.

Marker-vaccinated cattle

- group mates non-vaccinated 2.40×10^{-3} (1.23×10^{-3} - 4.39×10^{-3})

- whole group vaccinated 2.47×10^{-3} (1.27×10^{-3} - 4.51×10^{-3})

Non-vaccinated cattle 1.78×10^{-4} (8.38×10^{-5} - 8.01×10^{-4})

Therefore, importing one vaccinated cattle from a country not free from IBR would be associated with a 99.76% confidence of not introducing IBR into Switzerland under current risk management measures. This indicates that if 1000 animals were imported, the disease would be introduced on average on approx. 2 occasions. The difference between the import of a single vaccinated cattle in a group of non-vaccinated animals and the import of an entire group of vaccinated cattle is negligible. For the import of non-vaccinated cattle, the average value was 99.98%.

This represented a 13-fold higher risk for vaccinated animals than for non-vaccinated animals. Distributions for the output values are shown in Figures 21 and 22 as ascending cumulative frequency plots. They show the probability of the output being less than or equal to the x-axis value (Vose, 2003). In Figure 20 the output values are presented graphically.

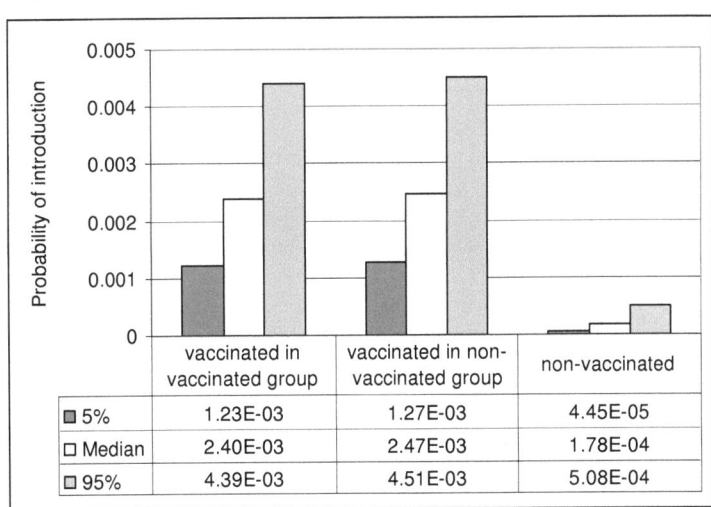

Figure 20. Obtained values for the probability of introduction of IBR into Switzerland by one single imported cattle

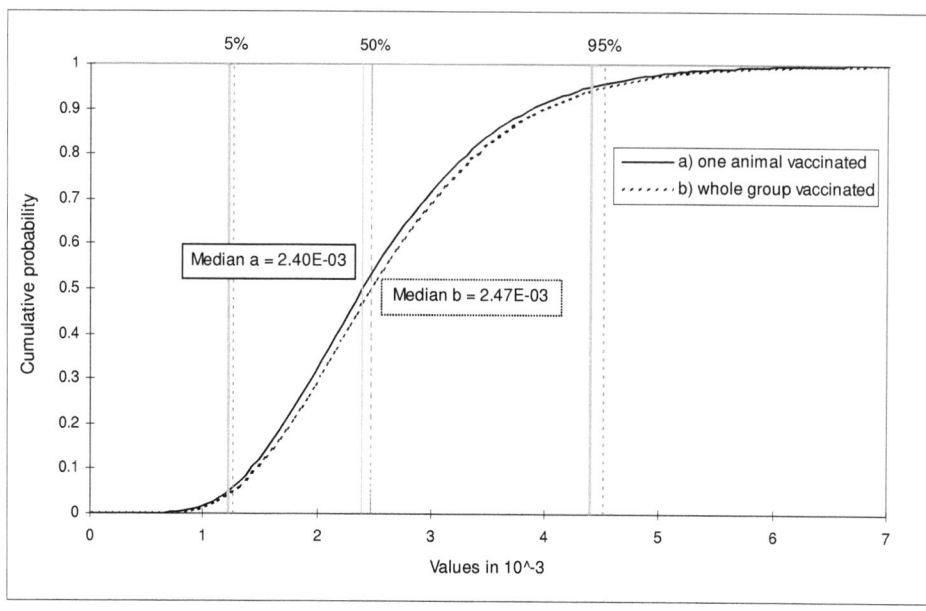

Figure 21. Cumulative distribution of the probability of IBR introduction in one vaccinated cattle

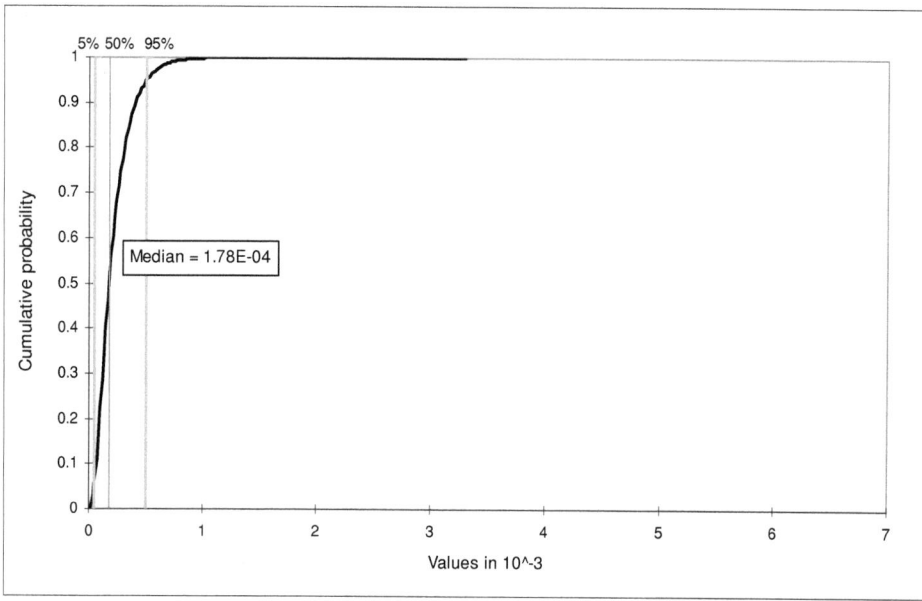

Figure 22. Cumulative distribution of the probability of IBR introduction in one non-vaccinated cattle

4.2. SENSITIVITY ANALYSIS

4.2.1. Aujeszky's disease

The tornado graph for the output value for a vaccinated pig is shown in Figure 23. Herd level prevalence in the exporting country had the largest effect on the output for vaccinated pigs. The number of days it took the animal to seroconvert against gE after infection was also important. These variables were all positively associated, i.e. if their value increased, the model output increased too. Similar impact had inherd prevalence in poorly protected herds, the proportion of herds being highly protected, the age of the animal, and transmission probability to a Swiss herd mate. Inherd prevalence and transmission probability were positively associated while the proportion of highly protected herds and the age of the pig were negatively associated. Smaller impact had inherd prevalence in highly protected herds, which was positively associated, and sensitivity of gE-ELISA, which was negatively associated. The probability of reactivation once in a lifetime in latently infected animals, the specificity of gE-ELISA, and the probability of clinical signs after reactivation had only a very small effect on the outcome.

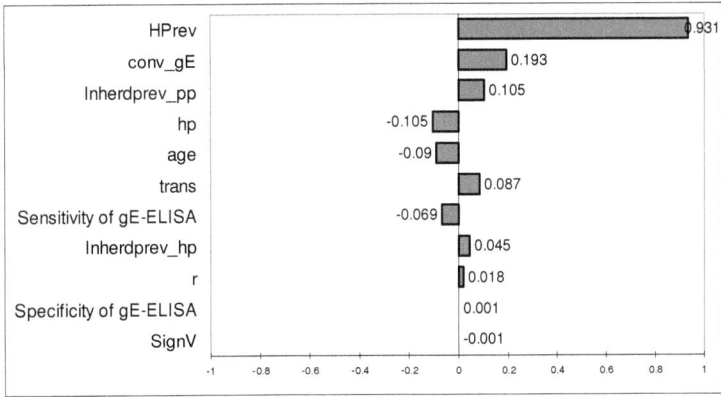

Figure 23. Regression sensitivity for a vaccinated pig (Standard b coefficient)

Figure 24 shows the tornado graph for the output value for a non-vaccinated pig. For non-vaccinated animals, too, herd level prevalence in the exporting country had the highest positively associated impact on the output. The second relevant input value was the probability of reactivation during separation in Switzerland, which was negatively associated. For a non-vaccinated pig, in contrast to the model for vaccinated pigs, test sensitivity was relevant as a negatively associated variable. Inherd prevalence and number of days until seroconversion had about the same positively associated impact, followed by the age of the animal at time of import with negative correlation. As for vaccinated animals, the probability of reactivation once in a lifetime in latently infected animals and test specificity had only a small effect on the outcome.

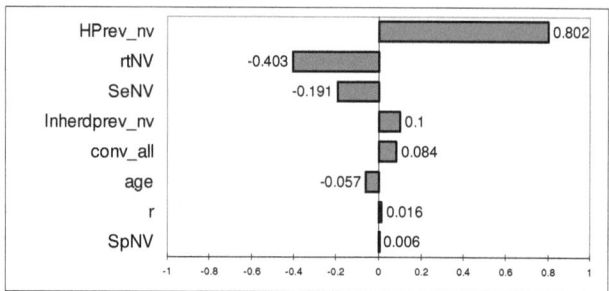

Figure 24. Regression sensitivity for a non-vaccinated pig (Standard b coefficient)

4.2.2. Infectious bovine rhinotracheitis

The tornado graph for vaccinated cattle is shown in Figure 25. Inherd prevalence in poorly protected herds and sensitivity of gE-ELISA had the highest impact on the output for vaccinated animals in a separation group with non-vaccinated animals. Inherd prevalence in poorly protected herds was positively associated while test sensitivity was negatively associated. A lower and approximately equal influence on the output resulted from the proportion of poorly protected herds, the probability of reactivation in separation in Switzerland, the incidence rate in the exporting country, and the sensitivity of test in Switzerland. Except for the probability of reactivation in separation, which was negatively associated, they were all positively associated with the model output. Transmission probability, specificity of indirect ELISA, and probability of reactivation at introduction into the Swiss herd had less impact on the model output. Again, reactivation probability was associated negatively while transmission probability and specificity of the test in Switzerland were positively associated. Probability of seroconversion, age of animals from age class 1, which were negatively associated, and reactivation once in a lifetime, which was positively associated, had a small effect. The number of group mates and days until seroconversion against gE had no effect.

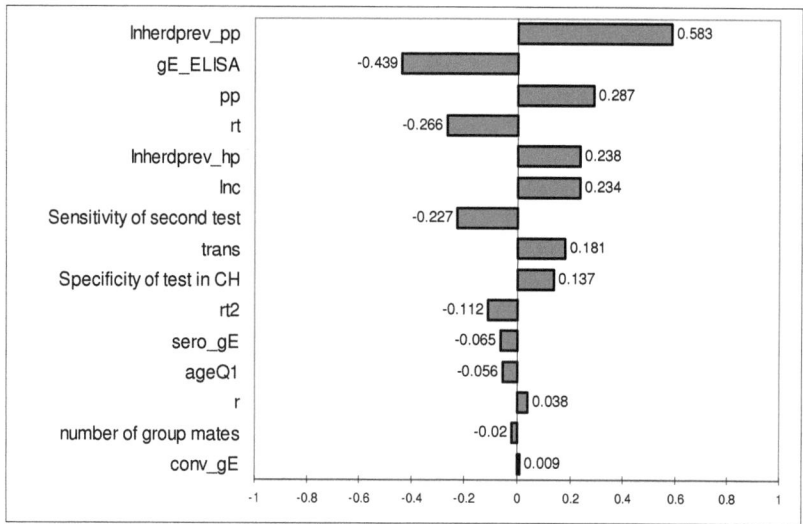

Figure 25. Regression sensitivity for a vaccinated cattle in a non-vaccinated group (Std b coeff)

80

For vaccinated animals in a separation group with vaccinated cattle, the sensitivity ranking was very similar to animals in a group of non-vaccinated cattle except for a reduced effect of reactivation at import. Furthermore, group sensitivity had a small effect on the output. Further details are therefore omitted but the tornado chart is shown in Figure 26.

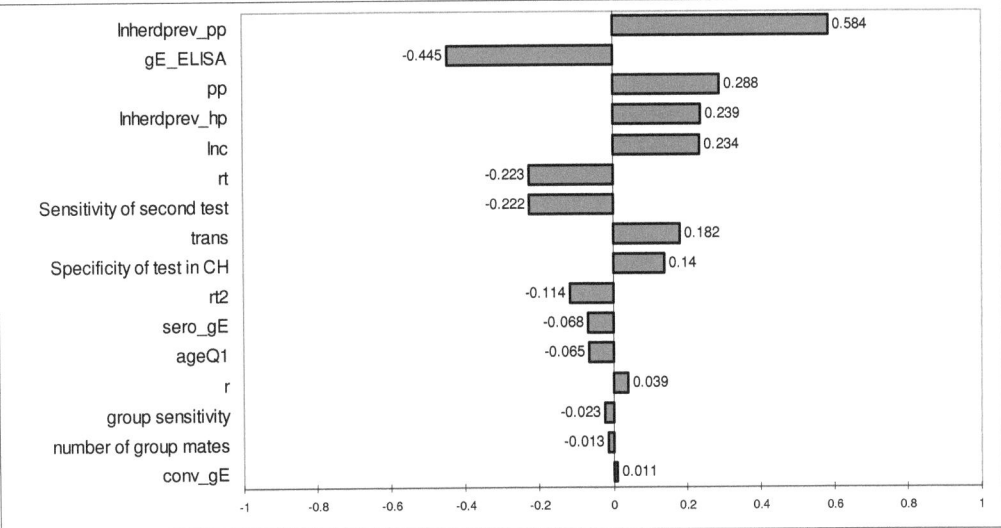

Figure 26. Regression sensitivity for a vaccinated cattle in a vaccinated group (Standard b coefficient)

For a non-vaccinated animal, the tornado chart is shown in Figure 28. For these animals, the sensitivity of gB-ELISA abroad was the most influential input variable with negative association. The probability of seroconversion as well as the sensitivity of the second test in Switzerland and the probability of reactivation in separation showed a strong negatively associated impact, followed by inherd prevalence and incidence in the exporting country with positive association. A smaller effect was observed for the following variables: probability of reactivation at introduction into Swiss herd, number of group mates in separation, test specificity, age of animal from age class 1, and transmission probability. While reactivation and number of group mates in separation as well as age for class 1 were negatively associated, the associations for test specificity and transmission probability were positive. Reactivation once in a lifetime and number of days until seroconversion had only a small effect on the model output.

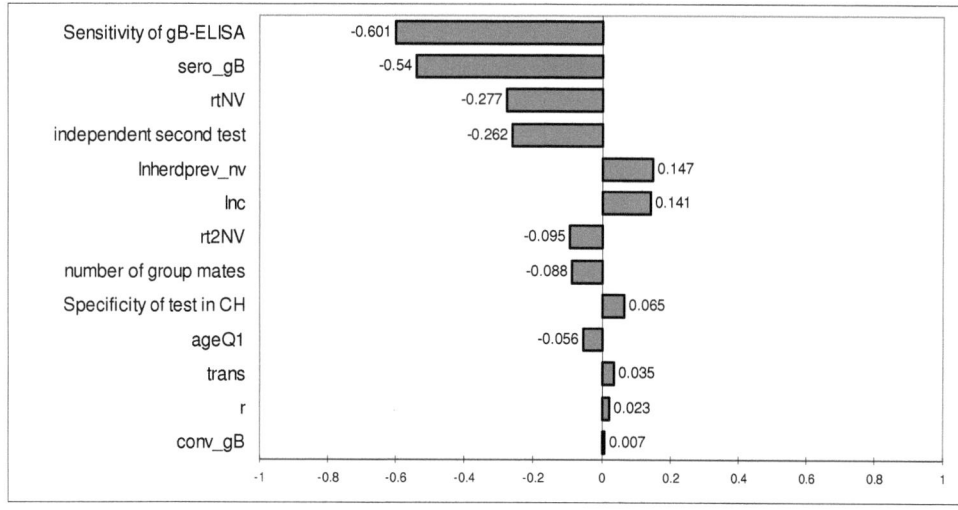

Figure 27. Regression sensitivity for a non-vaccinated cattle (Standard b coefficient)

Chapter 5   Discussion

5.1.   SOURCES OF INFORMATION FOR THE PRESENTED MODELS

Data from literature was used whenever possible to estimate model inputs, but great uncertainty existed, as it is difficult to extrapolate experimental data to the field or to apply results from one country or region to the population of another. Furthermore, for some parameters no literature data was available at all. We therefore decided to combine literature data with expert opinion.

We are aware that eliciting expert opinion after initially suggesting the values leads to a tendency to agree with the subjective opinion drawn from literature by the risk assessor. On the other hand, as shown by psychological research, human behaviour leads to bias in any case, especially when simply asking an individual to provide a probability. The methods of reasoning, or heuristics, employed when generating subjective estimates consistently introduces biases which can be quite large, regardless whether the individual is experienced in making estimates and is familiar with probability theory or is a novice in this field (Merkhofer and Keeney, 1987). Our eliciting process clearly avoids the individual's tendency to weight information, but the suggestion itself as made by the risk assessor may already be influenced by small unrepresentative sets of data with which he or she is familiar. Other sources of bias in the experts' estimates, but also already in the initial suggestion by the risk assessor, may be the human tendency to be overconfident and estimate uncertainty too narrowly, to resist changing one's mind in the face of new information, and to try to influence decisions and outcomes by casting beliefs in a particular direction. Nevertheless, our method of combining literature research with an expert consensus led to plausible estimates for our model inputs.

We opted for a small number of experts in order to enable a consensus process in estimating the values. With a large group of experts, this would have been impractical, and it would have been necessary to combine several estimates, which is a methodological problem in itself, although methods are described in the literature to derive distributions even from contrary expert opinions and to deal with many different estimates (Anonymous, 2004d). In the future, input values of these models can be changed as soon as further knowledge becomes available.

5.2.   MODELLING APPROACH

We consider the models to be a practicable and sound tool to conduct quantitative import risk assessments with regard to BoHV1 and AD introduction via marker-vaccinated animals. The models consider all relevant risk factors known to date and, although the models are characterised by a remarkable level of complexity, sufficient flexibility was maintained to enable translation to other infectious disease agents. Consequently, they are very useful to investigate possible existing and future import risks.

The weakness of both models is the unknown factor of herd prevalence in the exporting country. Since this had a strong influence but varies between different regions, no general statement can be made for an arbitrary animal from anywhere in Europe. However, both models allow the comparison between risks in vaccinated and non-vaccinated animals coming from a particular country or zone. A relative comparison was possible as long as the same herd level prevalences were assumed for vaccinated and non-vaccinated herds. With different herd level prevalences, as used for the AD model, the difference in herd level prevalences became the most effecting factor for the ratio between the results for a vaccinated and a non-vaccinated pig.

For the AD model, the Bayes model for sensitivity and specificity of gE-ELISA must be considered non-standard. In a next step, it could be useful to confirm the results by using a standard approach, such as WinBugs. On the other hand, the pooled estimator (sum of all true positives divided by sum of truly infected) yielded values for point estimate and variance estimate of sensitivity similar to the results of the Bayes model but within a smaller confidence interval. Additionally, it is questionable whether it is appropriate to use two different approaches to estimate sensitivity and specificity of gE-ELISA (Bayes model) and of PRV-ELISA (pert distribution). But since sensitivity analysis showed that test sensitivity had only a small effect on the outcome, there is no immediate need for further investigation.

The weakness of the IBR model is due to uncertainty factors related to test dependence, group size, and behaviour of the virus in mixed populations with vaccinated and non-vaccinated animals. The latter had only a small impact, but test dependence proved to be crucial for the output. Our approach to obtain an estimate for test dependence is rudimentary and certainly not a standard procedure. But since no further information was available, only a rough estimate could be produced that requires further investigation. To implement the model, it has to be clearly established which tests are used in Switzerland, because currently the indirect ELISA is used in Switzerland while for Europe, gB-ELISA is recommended by the EFSA. Therefore, under current procedures, there is no test dependence for non-vaccinated animals. However, the national reference laboratory is considering the adoption of European standards in the near future (Engels, M., Swiss reference laboratory for IBR, personal communication). This would require a change in model input for the second test, taking into account test dependence. Therefore, more research concerning test dependence would be of great benefit for obtaining more reliable results. For group sensitivities, the model might be too detailed, but the submodel for group sensitivity in separation was already available at SFVO, so we decided to include it into our model.

For both models, it would be helpful to have more information on the reactivation of latent infection over time, because sensitivity analysis showed a high impact for the values concerning reactivation at different points in the model. It is known that reactivation is possible and very likely to happen at some time in the life of a latently infected animal, but this knowledge is not sufficient to model precise probabilities for reactivation within given time periods between testing. However, no data on these aspects was available and the inputs are pure expert estimates.

5.2.1. Interpretation of the model outputs

All values discussed in this section are median values, and the values in brackets represent their 5th and 95th percentile, respectively.

The outputs obtained from our models can be interpreted in two ways. Firstly, they provide estimates for the probability of introduction of AD and IBR into Switzerland as defined in chapter 3. Secondly, they make it possible to compare the risks related to vaccinated and non-vaccinated animals. Because the output values are strongly influenced by the prevalence of infection in the exporting country, the quantitative estimates apply only to the individual situations in our example regions, Spain for AD and Saxony-Anhalt for IBR, respectively. But the ratio between the probabilities of introduction through vaccinated and non-vaccinated animals derived from the model is assumed to be applicable to other regions, too.

In the EFSA opinion on IBR-free animals and establishments, the AHAW panel concluded that because of the mentioned dependence on the *a-priori* probability of infection in the country of origin, there was no single definition of a BoHV-1 free animal. They recommended to determine an acceptable probability for an undetected infected animal and then combine the *a-priori* probability of infection with the quality parameters of the testing protocol to reach the defined threshold (Anonymous, 2005a). This is more or less what has been done in the presented model for IBR. The obtained results only apply to Saxony-Anhalt, but the model provides a tool to calculate estimates for any region as soon as the incidence in the area is known.

The results concerning AD and the import of live pigs from Spain showed for one vaccinated pig a 99.95% (99.99 - 99.84) probability of not introducing the disease. Even if this seems to be quite safe, the total number of imported animals needs to be considered. For example, if the number of imported animals is 100, average confidence decreases to 95.19% (99.42 - 85.24). Stated in different terms, if 100 pigs are imported annually, the disease would be introduced 5 times in 100 years. By contrast, for non-vaccinated pigs, confidence is nearly 100% (99.98 - 99.99995), and it would still be 99.99% for the import of 100 pigs. This indicates that when importing 100 non-vaccinated animals per year, the disease would be introduced on average less than once in a century.

For IBR, the probability was much higher than for AD. The main reasons are the higher prevalences used for IBR, the poorer test performances of the IBR ELISAs and the higher age of traded cattle compared to traded breeding pigs. For a single vaccinated cattle, average confidence was 99.76% (99.56 - 99.88); in other words, approx. 2 out of 1000 imported animals are infected and not detected by sanitary measures. For 100 animals, confidence decreases to 78.65% (64.39 - 88.41) on average, and for 1200 vaccinated cattle to only 5.60% (0.50 - 23.67). This means that on average, the disease would be introduced 21 times in 100 years if 100 animals are imported annually, and if 1200 vaccinated cattle are imported per year – as imported in 2005 – it would be almost certain for the disease to be introduced through at least one animal.

For non-vaccinated cattle, average confidence was 99.98% (99.95 - 99.996), indicating that roughly 2 out of 10'000 imported animals would introduce the disease. For the import of 100 animals, we can be 98.23% (94.98 - 99.56) confident of not introducing the disease, i.e. at an annual import rate of 100 animals, an undesired outcome would occur on average in 2 out of 100 years. For the import of 1200 non-vaccinated cattle from countries not free from disease, confidence is 80.74% (53.90 - 94.85), which means that at an annual import rate of 1200 cattle for 100 years, IBR would be introduced once every 5 years. These results clearly justify the targeting of Swiss establishments with imported animals in next year's annual risk-based national survey for IBR.

The AHAW panel recommends that an animal free from BoHV-1, unless coming from a free zone, should have a probability of at least 99.98% of not being infected. According to the report, this figure was obtained for a region with a prevalence of 10% by subjecting the animal to two tests, one at entry and one after at least 21 days of quarantine. However, the calculation did not take into account the probability of rare cases of animals that do not seroconvert and thus pose a risk for importing the infection. Furthermore, no dependence was assumed between the two tests (Anonymous, 2005b). The probability calculated with our model does not correspond exactly to the threshold recommended by the EFSA, because it also included reactivation probabilities, the testing scenario in Switzerland after import, and the probability of transmission to a Swiss herd mate. Nevertheless, the results should be roughly in the same range because in both cases, the animals are tested twice and the results depend on the prevalence in the exporting country and on test performance.

Our model showed exactly the required 99.98% for the probability of the animal not harbouring BoHV-1 when separation after import is suspended. But if we change the input values for the model according to the assumptions made in the EFSA report, assuming a probability of seroconversion of 100% and independence between tests, we obtain similar probabilities. Should the EU adopt the EFSA recommendations and require two tests during quarantine abroad, a probability of 99.992% or greater could be reached provided that testing after import in Switzerland is continued. The model shows that currently, cattle arriving at the Swiss border from countries not free from IBR after undergoing one test in quarantine do not meet the recommended criterion of a 99.98% probability of not being infected. Only additional measures applied in Switzerland during separation can provide a sufficient probability of not introducing the infection.

The finding that vaccinated animals generally represent a higher risk of introducing the disease than non-vaccinated animals is consistent with other findings in modelling and risk assessment. Graat et al. (2001) found the vaccination status to be the strongest factor for modelling R_0 between herds in an IBR surveillance programme, and the scientific report by the EFSA also documents a lower probability of disease freedom for vaccinated animals (Anonymous, 2005b). The differences are due to the lower test performance of the gE-ELISAs, the lower probability of clinical signs in vaccinated animals, and the lower reactivation and transmission rates.

5.2.2. Sensitivity analysis

Understanding how the output is affected by the model's input variables is useful for analysing the results and refining the model if appropriate. Variables with large impact on the outcome can be revalidated and adjusted while variables that have only a small impact may be neglected. @RISK offers comprehensive statistical report options to facilitate result interpretation as well as graphical illustration capabilities. We used tornado charts to conduct our sensitivity analysis.

Tornado charts based on step-wise regression as presented in section 4.2 must be interpreted with caution. Since they illustrate the degree to which the uncertainty of the output is affected by the uncertainty of the individual variables, they do not account for fixed parameters that may also affect the results. The impact of parameters with only a small variation might be underestimated as well. Step-wise regression is performed for each input value using the data obtained from the iterations. Only large differences in coefficients indicate greater or smaller effects, whereas for input values with similar coefficients, the ranking might change for each simulation (@RISK manual). Additionally, it makes sense to limit the number of variables represented in the plot (Vose, 2003).

In both models, presence of the disease in the exporting country as well as in the establishment of origin (inherd prevalence / proportion of highly protected vaccinated herds) had an effect on the output. This means that a higher disease prevalence in the exporting country increases the probability of introduction in imported animals irrespective of test performance. This finding is consistent with the opinion published by the AHAW panel (Anonymous, 2005a).

For AD, herd level prevalence was the most important input value. Since we chose different inputs for vaccinated and non-vaccinated herds, there was a large difference between the outputs for a vaccinated and a non-vaccinated pig. By using the same herd level prevalence for both types of herds, the probability of introduction for vaccinated animals was only 2.9-fold higher than for non-vaccinated animals, which is more consistent with the ratio obtained for vaccinated and non-vaccinated cattle in the IBR model. On the other hand, it seemed reasonable to interpret the data differently for vaccinated and non-vaccinated herds, as an outbreak of clinical disease after the introduction of PRV is very likely in non-vaccinated seronegative herds. We regard the occurrence of clinical symptoms as an additional possible detection method for non-vaccinated herds and therefore assume a smaller prevalence of infected but not detected herds than in vaccinated ones.

Since pigs are only tested once for AD, which is during separation abroad, the question whether the animal has already seroconverted at time of testing had an important effect on the outcome for a vaccinated pig. A newly infected pig that would seroconvert later will not be detected. As a consequence, the number of days until seroconversion was highly positively associated. The longer it takes for the animal to seroconvert, the higher the chance that it will be tested before seroconversion. For non-vaccinated animals, time until seroconversion is shorter than for vaccinated animals, therefore, fewer animals are likely to be tested before seroconversion, and the probability of seroconversion had a smaller effect than in the model for vaccinated pigs. As we used the estimated age of the pig to calculate the probability of seroconversion, it was not surprising that age had also an effect on the output. It was negatively associated, which can be explained by the fact that the calculation for the daily risk of infection was derived from dividing one by age. It followed that, the younger the pig, the larger was its daily risk of infection.

For a non-vaccinated pig, the probability of reactivation of a latent infection during separation in Switzerland was crucial because the probability of clinical signs after reactivation was always 100% and would lead to detection of the infected animal. It was strongly negatively associated, indicating that the higher the probability of reactivation at import, the higher the probability of detecting the infection by clinical signs during separation and therefore the smaller the probability of introducing AD into Switzerland (model output). On the other hand, for vaccinated animals, the role of reactivation at import was negligible as clinical signs are very unlikely. However, the probability of clinical signs, even when very small, had a negatively associated effect on disease detection and therefore on model output. The effects of reactivation once in a lifetime and of test specificity was very small due to their narrow ranges and their large values close to 100%.

Test sensitivity also affected the output of the AD model. It was larger for non-vaccinated animals, which may be due to the wider range in the input for sensitivity of PRV-ELISA compared to the values derived from the Bayes model. As expected, the correlation was negative. Since virus excretion is reduced in vaccinated pigs, virus transmission to its Swiss herd mates had some positively associated effect on the output as well. For a non-vaccinated pig, virus transmission was estimated to be 100%, indicating that only reactivation affected the output whereas transmission was certain to occur once the infection has been reactivated.

For the IBR model, we used the same input data for disease presence in the exporting country for vaccinated and non-vaccinated herds, mainly because more detailed information was not available. As a result, incidence as a basis to calculate herd prevalence had a smaller effect on the IBR model than herd prevalence for AD. This might be one reason why the differences in the probabilities of introduction between vaccinated and non-vaccinated cattle are quite small. The use of the same incidence values for vaccinated and non-vaccinated herds is subject to the same critical arguments as mentioned above with respect to AD.

The much more complicated import scenario for cattle with several tests performed on the animal explains the importance of the different test performance input values. Test sensitivity was one of the factors with the largest effects in the IBR model. The sensitivity of the second test was also crucial since the test performed in Switzerland must be regarded as dependent to some extent. On the other hand, the probability of animals not seroconverting affected the model output because these animals cannot be detected by testing. Obviously, since a detected animal does not introduce the disease, all inputs that affect the detection probability of an animal are negatively associated.

For group sensitivity in separation and in sentinel animals, the probability of reactivation during separation and at introduction into a Swiss herd and the probability of virus transmission as well as the number of group mates are important. Reactivation was negatively associated since the detection probability increases if the animal infects its group mates. On the other hand, transmission probability was positively associated, indicating that transmission to Swiss herd mates makes disease introduction more likely. We regard the lower probability of reactivation and of virus transmission as one of the main reasons for the differences in model output for vaccinated and non-vaccinated cattle.

Additionally, reactivation during separation also had an effect on the model since we considered animals with a reactivated infection as serologically different from before and assumed full test sensitivity again for a second test. Because the sentinel animals represented the last opportunity to detect the disease, the specificity of the sentinel test had some effect if no virus is transmitted to the sentinels. Thus, a false positive result would prompt further investigation not only in sentinels but also in the imported animal. The higher the specificity, the lower the chance to detect the infected animal accidentally due to a false negative result in a sentinel animal. It was therefore positively associated. The probability of reactivation once in a lifetime and the number of days until seroconversion had only a very small effect on the model output.

5.2.3. Different scenarios

For the import of pigs, additional sanitary measures are easy to implement. The animals are so far only tested once but kept in separation in Switzerland, including blood sampling for other diseases. To obtain greater confidence when importing vaccinated animals, a second test could be performed in Switzerland. By introducing test sensitivity rather than probability of clinical signs in vaccinated animals into the model, the chance of detecting a latently infected animal increased and confidence could be improved to 99.996% (99.987 - 99.9997), which comes close to the safety level for a non-vaccinated pig. Assuming the same herd level prevalence for vaccinated and non-vaccinated herds, the probability of introducing the infection became even lower for vaccinated animals than for non-vaccinated animals if a second test was performed on the vaccinated ones. This underscores to the large effect of disease presence in the exporting country, which requires thorough consideration before import regulations are devised.

For IBR, many measures have already been implemented, and it is difficult to imagine additional useful test methods. Because of test dependence, performing a third test on the animal itself would not yield much more information. On the other hand, testing sentinel animals may not be very helpful in detecting latently infected vaccinated animals because they are not very likely to reactivate the infection or to transmit virus after reactivation. In the case of vaccinated animals, one possible suggestion is therefore to retest the animal itself by a third test after a reasonable interval instead of testing sentinel animals.

Another possibility to detect latent infection in vaccinated (and non-vaccinated) animals would be a treatment with dexamethasone to reactivate infection, followed by virus isolation from nasal swabs. However, this scenario appears not very practicable because it would require isolation throughout the test period, which is expensive. Moreover, the scenario is questionable for medical and animal welfare reasons.

Since transmission probability and group sensitivity in separation affected the model output, we calculated the output in case of one vaccinated animal within a non-vaccinated separation group and, additionally, for the situation of a whole group of imported vaccinated animals. Animals imported in groups of vaccinated cattle have a slightly higher probability of introducing the disease, but the differences between outputs were minimal.

5.3. RECOMMENDATIONS FOR DECISION-MAKERS

Results of our models do not justify the recommendation of the import of pigs that are marker-vaccinated against AD. Since the results were strongly dependent on herd level prevalence in the exporting country, solutions should be found to deal with this issue. It may not be sensible to divide exporting countries merely into free and not free. It should be considered whether it is legally possible to differentiate infected countries on the basis of actual prevalences. Thereafter, cut-off values for herd level prevalence could be defined using the presented models. Should the import of vaccinated animals appear desirable under such circumstances, a second gE-ELISA during separation in Switzerland is strongly recommended. Other possible methods to reduce the risk might be a prolonged quarantine abroad for vaccinated animals. Since in our model the exporting country tested its herds every four months, requirements for further herd testing do not seem reasonable. However, restrictions concerning sample size or time after the last test in the establishment of origin may further decrease the risk.

For IBR, the differences between the probabilities of introducing the disease through vaccinated and non-vaccinated animals are not as large as for AD but large enough to justify import restrictions on vaccinated animals. This is consistent with the recommendations in the EFSA opinion (Anonymous, 2005a). However, it must be kept in mind that our model assumed the same herd level prevalence for vaccinated and non-vaccinated herds, which might not be realistic. The same arguments as outlined above for pig herds, albeit with a smaller impact, must be considered with regard to the risk of not detecting a newly infected herd.

New requirements for pre-shipment testing in the exporting country should be implemented as recommended by the EFSA, because under the current protocol, animals do not attain the necessary 99.98% probability of not being infected at shipment. In quarantine, two tests should be performed on the animals, one at entry and one after at least 21 days (Anonymous, 2005b). However, to obtain more reliable results, the values for test dependence and the probabilities of reactivation at different stages need to be further investigated and validated.

References

Ackermann, M., Muller, H.K., Bruckner, L., Riggenbach, C., Kihm, U., 1989; The control of infectious bovine rhinotracheitis (IBR) in Switzerland from 1978 to 1988. Schweiz Arch Tierheilkd 131, 397-407.

Ackermann, Muller, H. K., Bruckner, L., Kihm, U, 1990a; Eradication of infectious bovine rhinotracheitis in Switzerland: review and prospects. Vet Microbiol 23, 365-370.

Ackermann, M., Weber, H.P., Wyler, R., 1990b; Aspects of infectious bovine rhinotracheitis eradication programmes in a fattening cattle farm. Prev Vet Med 9, 121-130.

Ackermann, M., Engels M., 2003; Kapitel Herpesviren, Aujeszkysche Krankheit. In: Beilagen zur Vorlesung Virologie 2003/2004, Teil I, Virus Portraits, p.50-55.

Ackermann, M., Engels, M., 2006; Pro and contra IBR-eradication. Vet Microbiol 113, 293-302.

Anonymous, 1997, IBR control porgammes, Maastricht, 26-27 June 1997 (P. Franken, Ed.); Animal Health Service, Deventer, The Netherlands.

Anonymous, 1998; Agreement on the application of sanitary and phytosanitary measures. The WTO Agreement Series No. 4 (Geneva, WTO), p. 49.

Anonymous, 2002; Basic principles for risk analyses conducted at the Swiss federal veterinary office (Bern, SFVO), www.bvet.admin.ch

Anonymous, 2004a; Additional guarantees for intra-Community trade in bovine animals relating to infectious bovine rhinotracheitis and the approval of the eradication programmes presented by certain member states (Brussels, EU Commission)

Anonymous, 2004b; BHV1-Verordnung: Neufassung vom 3.11.2004 der Verordnung zum Schutz der Rinder vor einer Infektion mit dem bovinen Herpesvirus Typ I (BHV1-VO) vom 5.11.1997 (Berlin)

Anonymous, 2004c; Handbook on import risk analysis for animals and animal products: Introduction and qualitative risk analysis (Paris, OIE).

Anonymous, 2004d; Handbook on import risk analysis for animals and animal products: Quantitative risk assessment (Paris, OIE).

Anonymous, 2004e; Importregelungen zum Import von lebenden Tieren der Schweinegattung in die Schweiz (Bern, SFVO). www.bvet.admin.ch

Anonymous, 2005a; AHAW Opinion: Definition of a BoHV-1-free animal and a BoHV-1-free holding, and the procedures to verify and maintain this status (Parma, EFSA, AHAW Panel).

Anonymous, 2005b; AHAW Report: Definition of a BoHV-1-free animal and a BoHV-1-free holding, and the procedures to verify and maintain this status (Parma, EFSA, AHAW Panel).

Anonymous, 2005c; Cahier des charges technique du système national d'appellation de cheptel en matière de rhinotracheite infectieuse bovine (Paris, ACERSA).

Anonymous, 2005d; Importregelungen zum Import von lebenden Tieren der Rindergattung in die Schweiz (Bern, SFVO). www.bvet.admin.ch

Anonymous, 2005e; OIE Terrestrial animal health code, 14th edition (Paris, OIE). http://www.oie.int

Arias, M., Moyano, M., Escribano, J.M., Sanchez-Vizcaino, J.M., 1992, Evaluation of two ELISA kits for the detection of Aujeszky's disease antibodies in pigs. Vet Rec 131, 391-393.

Austin, C.C., Weigel, R.M., Hungerford, L.L., Biehl, L.R.G., 1993; Factors affecting the risk of infection with pseudorabies virus in Illinois swine herds. Prev Vet Med 17, 161-173.

Babiuk, L.A., 2002; Vaccination: a management tool in veterinary medicine. Vet J 164, 188-201.

Bech-Nielsen, S., Miller, G.Y., Bowman, G.L., Burkholder, R.H., Dodaro, S.J., Palte, W.J., 1995; Risk factors identified as source of new infections (area spread) with pseudorabies (Aujeszky's disease) virus in 50 swine herds in a continous geographical area of Ohio. Prev Vet Med 23, 53-64.

Beer, M., Konig, P., Schielke, G., Trapp, S., 2003; Diagnostic markers in the prevention of bovine herpesvirus type 1: possibilities and limitations. Berl Munch Tierarztl Wochenschr 116, 183-191.

Beer, M., Mettenleiter, T.C., 2004; DIVA - die moderne Art der Tierseuchenbekämpfung. Tierarztl Umschau 59, 551 - 559.

Boelaert, F., Deluyker, H., Maes, D., Godfroid, J., Raskin, A., Varewijck, H., Pensaert, M., Nauwynck, H., Castryck, F., Miry, C., Robijns, J.M., Hoet, B., Segers, E., Van Vlaenderen, I., Robert, A., Koenen, F., 1999; Prevalence of herds with young sows seropositive to pseudorabies (Aujeszky's disease) in northern Belgium. Prev Vet Med 41, 239-255.

Boelaert, F., Speybroeck, N., de Kruif, A., Aerts, M., Burzykowski, T., Molenberghs, G., Berkvens, D.L., 2005; Risk factors for bovine herpesvirus-1 seropositivity. Prev Vet Med 69, 285-295.

Bosch, J.C., de Jong, M.C.M., Maissan, J., van Oirschot, J.T. 1997; Quantification of experimental transmission of bovine herpes-virus 1 in cattle vaccinated with marker vaccines. Bovine Practitioner, pp. 49-50.

Bosch, J.C., De Jong, M.C., Franken, P., Frankena, K., Hage, J.J., Kaashoek, M.J., Maris-Veldhuis, M.A., Noordhuizen, J.P., Van der Poel, W.H., Verhoeff, J., Weerdmeester, K., Zimmer, G.M., Van Oirschot, J.T., 1998; An inactivated gE-negative marker vaccine and an experimental gD-subunit vaccine reduce the incidence of bovine herpesvirus 1 infections in the field. Vaccine 16, 265-271.

Bouma, A., De Smit, A.J., De Jong, M.C.M., De Kluijver, E.P., Moormann, R.J.M., 2000; Determination of the onset of the herd-immunity induced by the E2 sub-unit vaccine against classical swine fever virus. Vaccine 18, 1374-1381.

Breidenbach, E., Hauser, R., Stark, K., 2004; Performance of risk analysis at the Federal veterinary office. Berl Munch Tierarztl 117, 171-176.

Cameron, A., Martin, T., 2003; The use of scenario-tree modelling using multiple complex data sources to demonstrate Danish freedom from classical swine fever. ISVEE, Viña del Mar, Chile, November 2003.

Cocker, F.M., Gaskell, R.M., Newby, T.J., Gaskell, C.J., Stokes, C.R., Bourne, F.J., 1984; Efficacy of early (48 and 96 hour) protection against feline viral rhinotracheitis following intranasal vaccination with a live temperature sensitive mutant. Vet Rec 114, 353-354.

Covello, V.T., Merkhofer, M.W., 1993; Risk assessment methods: Approaches for assessing health and environmental risks. Plenum Publishing, New York.

de Jong, M., Diekmann, O., 1992; A method to calculate - for computer-simulated infections - the threshold value R that predicts whether or not the infection will spread. Prev Vet Med 12, 269-285.

de Jong, M., Kimman, T.G., 1994; Experimental quantification of vaccine-induced reduction in virus transmission. Vaccine 12, 761-766.

de Jong, M., 1995; Mathematical modelling in veterinary epidemiology: why model building is important. Prev Vet Med 25, 183 - 193.

de Leeuw, P.W., van Oirschot, J.T., 1985; Vaccines against Aujeszky's disease: evaluation of their efficacy under standardized laboratory conditions. Vet Q 7, 191-197.

Denzin, N., Ewert, B. 2005; Stand der BHV 1-Tilgung in Sachsen-Anhalt. 5. Internationales Symposium zur BHV 1-, BVD- und Paratuberkulose-Bekämpfung (Stedal, Germany)

Dispas, M., Lemaire, M., Speybroeck, N., Berkvens, D., Schreiber, P., Vanopdenbosch, E., Thiry, E., Kerkhofs, P., 2003; Study of risk factors for the transmission of bovine herpesvirus-1 according to the farm production type. Scientific Report 2001 - 2002 of the Veterinary and Agrochemical Research Center, p.17-19.

Durham, P.J., Sillars, H.M., Hobbs, I.F., 1985; Comparison of the enzyme-linked immunosorbent assay (ELISA) and serum neutralisation test for the serodiagnosis of Aujeszky's disease. New Zeal Vet J 33, 132-135.

Ehrensperger, F., Kihm, U., Probst, U., Irrall, B., 1984; Epidemiology of Aujeszky's disease in Switzerland. Schweiz Arch Tierheilkd 126 (8), 429-439.

Eloit, M., Fargeaud, D., Vannier, P., Toma, B., 1989; Development of an ELISA to differentiate between animals either vaccinated with or infected by Aujeszky's disease virus. Vet Rec 124, 91-94.

Engels, M., Giuliani, C., Wild, P., Beck, T.M., Loepfe, E., Wyler, R., 1986; The genome of bovine herpesvirus 1 (BHV-1) strains exhibiting a neuropathogenic potential compared to known BHV-1 strains by restriction site mapping and cross-hybridization. Virus Res 6, 57-73.

Engels, M., Ackermann, M., 1996; Pathogenesis of ruminant herpesvirus infections. Vet Microbiol 53, 3-15.

Ferrari, M., Brack, A., Romanelli, M.G., Mettenleiter, T.C., Corradi, A., Dal Mas, N., Losio, M.N., Silini, R., Pinoni, C., Pratelli, A., 2000; A study of the ability of a TK-negative and gI/gE-negative pseudorabies virus (PRV) mutant inoculated by different routes to protect pigs against PRV infection. J Vet Med B Infect Dis Vet Public Health 47, 753-762.

Flint, S.J., Enquist, L.W., Skalka, A.M., 2003; Principles of virology, Vol 1, Second edition. Blackwell Publishing, Oxford.

Graat, E.A., de Jong, M.C., Frankena, K., Franken, P., 2001; Modelling the effect of surveillance programmes on spread of bovine herpesvirus 1 between certified cattle herds. Vet Microbiol 79, 193-208.

Grant, R.H., Scheidt, A.B., Rueff, L.R., 1994; Aerosol transmission of a viable virus affecting swine: explanation of an epizootic of pseudorabies. Int J Biometeorol 38, 33-39.

Hadorn, D., Hauser, R., Stark, K.D., 2002a; Epidemiological basis and results of the National Survey 2001 conducted in the Swiss pig population. Schweiz Arch Tierheilkd 144 (10), 532-541.

Hadorn, D. C., Rufenacht, J., Hauser, R., Stark, K.D., 2002b; Risk-based design of repeated surveys for the documentation of freedom from non-highly contagious diseases. Prev Vet Med 56 (3), 179-192.

Hage, J.J., Schukken, Y.H., Barkema, H.W., Benedictus, G., Rijsewijk, F.A., Wentink, G.H., 1996, Population dynamics of bovine herpesvirus 1 infection in a dairy herd. Vet Microbiol 53, 169-180.

Hage, J.J., Vellema, P., Schukken, Y.H., Barkema, H.W., Rijsewijk, F.A., van Oirschot, J.T., Wentink, G.H., 1997; Sheep do not have a major role in bovine herpesvirus 1 transmission. Vet Microbiol 57, 41-54.

Hahn, G., Jarosch, M., Wang, J.B., Berbes, C., McVoy, M.A., 2003; Tn7-mediated introduction of DNA sequences into bacmid-cloned cytomegalovirus genomes for rapid recombinant virus construction. J Virol Methods 107, 185-194.

Hathaway, S.C., 1991; The application of risk assessment methods in making veterinary public health and animal health decisions. Rev Sci Tech OIE 10, 215-231.

Hauser, R., Breidenbach, E., Thur, B., Griot, C., Engels, M., Stark, K., 2004; Import risk analysis in animal disease control. Berl Munch Tierarztl 117, 188-192.

Henderson, L.M., 2005; Overview of marker vaccine and differential diagnostic test technology. Biologicals 33, 203-209.

Hofmann-Lehmann, R., Meli, M.L., Dreher, U. M., Gonczi, E., Deplazes, P., Braun, U., Engels, M., Schupbach, J., Jorger, K., Thoma, R., Griot, C., Stark, K.D., Willi, B., Schmidt, J., Kocan, K. M., Lutz, H., 2004; Concurrent infections with vector-borne pathogens associated with fatal hemolytic anemia in a cattle herd in Switzerland. J Clin Microbiol 42 (8), 3775-3780.

Jacobs, L., Voets, R., Bianchi, A.T.J., 1999; Detection of pseudorabies virus DNA in individual single-reactor pigs found in certified pseudorabies-free herds. Res Vet Sci 67, 305-307.

Kaashoek, M.J., van Oirschot, J.T., 1996; Early immunity induced by a live gE-negative bovine herpesvirus 1 marker vaccine. Vet Microbiol 53, 191-197.

Kit, S., Sheppard, M., Ichimura, H., Kit, M., 1987; Second-generation pseudorabies virus vaccine with deletions in thymidine kinase and glycoprotein genes. Am J Vet Res 48, 780-793.

Knopf, L., Reist, M., Breidenbach, E. 2004; Abschätzung der Wahrscheinlichkeit für das Einschleppen von IBR/IPV, EBL, Brucellose der Schafe und Ziegen und Aujeszky'scher Krankheit in die Schweiz (Bern, SFVO). www.bvet.admin.ch

Konig, P., Beer, M., Makoschey, B., Teifke, J.P., Polster, U., Giesow, K., Keil, G.M., 2003; Recombinant virus-expressed bovine cytokines do not improve efficacy of a bovine herpesvirus 1 marker vaccine strain. Vaccine 22, 202-212.

Koeppel, C., Knopf, L., Ryser, M.-P., Miserez, R., Thür, B., Stärk, K., 2006; Sero-surveillance for selected infectious disease agents in wild boars (Sus scrofa) and outdoor pigs in Switzerland. Eur J Wildl Res (in press).

Kramps, J.A., Banks, M., Beer, M., Kerkhofs, P., Perrin, M., Wellenberg, G.J., Oirschot, J.T., 2004; Evaluation of tests for antibodies against bovine herpesvirus 1 performed in national reference laboratories in Europe. Vet Microbiol 102, 169-181.

Kupferschmied, H.U., Kihm, U., Bachmann, P., Muller, K.H., Ackermann, M., 1986; Transmission of IBR/IPV virus in bovine semen: A case report. Theriogenology 25, 439-443.

Lake, D.E., Hutchings, C.R., Aalders, N.G., 1990; Aujeszky's disease in dogs - more confirmed cases. Surveillance 17, 24.

Lemaire, M., Weynants, V., Godfroid, J., Schynts, F., Meyer, G., Letesson, J.J., Thiry, E., 2000a; Effects of bovine herpesvirus type 1 infection in calves with maternal antibodies on immune response and virus latency. J Clin Microbiol 38, 1885-1894.

Lemaire, M., Meyer, G., Baranowski, E., Schynts, F., Wellemans, G., Kerkhofs, P., Thiry, E., 2000b; Production of bovine herpesvirus type 1-seronegative latent carriers by administration of a live-attenuated vaccine in passively immunized calves. J Clin Microbiol 38, 4233-4238.

Leontides, L., Ewald, C., Mortensen, S., Willeberg, P., 1994a; Factors associated with circulation of Aujeszkys disease virus in fattening herds of an intensively vaccinated area of Northern Germany. Prev Vet Med 20, 63-78.

Leontides, L., Ewald, C., Willeberg, P., 1994b; Herd risk-factors for serological evidence of Aujeszkys disease virus infection of breeding sows in Northern Germany (1990-1991). J Vet Med B Infect Dis Vet Public Health 41, 554-560.

Leontides, L., Ewald, C., Mortensen, S., Willeberg, P., 1995; Factors associated with the seroprevalence of Aujeszkys disease virus in seropositive breeding herds of Northern Germany during area-wide compulsory vaccination. Prev Vet Med 23, 73-85.

Liess, B., 1997; Virusinfektionen einheimischer Haussäugetiere - Ein Leitfaden zur klinischen Veterinärvirologie, Vol 1. Enke Verlag, Hannover.

Ludwig, H., 1983; Bovine herpesvirus type 1, In: Roizman, B., The herpesviruses. Plenum Press, New York, pp. 135-214.

MacDiarmid, S.C., 1990; An Aujeszky's disease eradication program for New Zealand. Surveillance 17, 20-22.

Maes, D., Deluyker, H., Verdonck, M., Castryck, F., Miry, C., Vrijens, B., de Kruif, A., 2000; Herd factors associated with the seroprevalences of four major respiratory pathogens in slaughter pigs from farrow-to-finish pig herds. Vet Res 31, 313-327.

Magana-Urbina, A., Solorio Rivera, J.L., Segura-Correa, J.C., 2005; Infectious bovine rhinotracheitis in dairy herds in the Cotzio-Tejaro region of Michoacan, Mexico. Tec Pecu Mex 43, 27-37.

Makoschey, B., Keil, G.M., 2000; Early immunity induced by a glycoprotein E-negative vaccine for infectious bovine rhinotracheitis. Vet Rec 147, 189-191.

Makoschey, B., Lütticken, D., 2002; Markierte Impfstoffe und Diagnostika. Amtstierärztlicher Dienst und Lebensmittelkontrolle 2002, 144-148.

Mars, M.H., de Jong, M.C.M., van Maanen, C., Hage, J.J., van Oirschot, J.T., 2000; Airborne transmission of bovine herpesvirus 1 infections in calves under field conditions. Vet Microbiol 76, 1-13.

Martin, T., Cameron, A. 2006; Evaluation of complex surveillance systems. In: Text book to SAFOSO and AusVet course (Bern).

Mellencamp, M.W., Pfeiffer, N.E., Suiter, B.T., Harness, J.R., Beckenhauer, W.H., 1989; Identification of pseudorabies virus-exposed swine with a gI glycoprotein enzyme-linked immunosorbent assay. J Clin Microbiol 27, 2208-2213.

Mengeling, W.L., Lager, K.M., Volz, D.M., Brockmeier, S.L., 1992; Effect of various vaccination procedures on shedding, latency, and reactivation of attenuated and virulent pseudorabies virus in swine. Am J Vet Res 53, 2164-2173.

Merkhofer, M.W., Keeney, R.L., 1987; A multiattribute utility analysis of alternative sites for the disposal of nuclear waste. Risk Anal 7, 173-194.

Mettenleiter, T.C., 1995; Progress in the development of vaccines against Aujeszky's disease. Tierarztl Prax 23, 570-574.

Mettenleiter, T.C., 2000; Aujeszky's disease (pseudorabies) virus: the virus and molecular pathogenesis - state of the art, June 1999. Vet Res 31, 99-115.

Meyers, G., Saalmuller, A., Buttner, M., 1999; Mutations abrogating the RNase activity in glycoprotein E(rns) of the pestivirus classical swine fever virus lead to virus attenuation. J Virol 73, 10224-10235.

Mollema, L., Rijsewijk, F.A., Nodelijk, G., de Jong, M.C., 2005; Quantification of the transmission of bovine herpesvirus 1 among red deer (Cervus elaphus) under experimental conditions. Vet Microbiol 111, 25-34.

Moormann, R.J., de Rover, T., Briaire, J., Peeters, B.P., Gielkens, A.L., van Oirschot, J.T., 1990; Inactivation of the thymidine kinase gene of a gI deletion mutant of pseudorabies virus generates a safe but still highly immunogenic vaccine strain. J Gen Virol 71 (Pt 7), 1591-1595.

Moormann, R.J., Bouma, A., Kramps, J.A., Terpstra, C., De Smit, H.J., 2000; Development of a classical swine fever subunit marker vaccine and companion diagnostic test. Vet Microbiol 73, 209-219.

Moraes, M.P., Chinsangaram, J., Brum, M.C., Grubman, M.J., 2003; Immediate protection of swine from foot-and-mouth disease: a combination of adenoviruses expressing interferon alpha and a foot-and-mouth disease virus subunit vaccine. Vaccine 22, 268-279.

Motha, M.X.J., Eernisse, K.A., 1992; Comparison of three glycoprotein-I-ELISAs for Aujeszky's disease virus. Vet Rec 130, 593-540.

Muller, T., Klupp, B., Zellmer, R., Teuffert, J., Ziedler, K., Possardt, C., Mewes, L., Dresenkamp, B., Conraths, F.J., Mettenleiter, T.C., 1998a; Characterisation of pseudorabies virus isolated from wild boar (Sus scrofa). Vet Rec 143, 337-340.

Muller, T., Teuffert, J., Ziedler, K., Possardt, C., Kramer, M., Staubach, C., Conraths, F.J., 1998b; Pseudorabies in the European wild boar from Eastern Germany. J Wildl Dis 34, 251-258.

Muller, T., Conraths, F.J., Hahn, E.C., 2000; Pseudorabies virus infection (Aujeszky's disease) in wild swine. Infect Dis Rev 2, 27-34.

Pastoret, P.P., Babiuk, L.A., Misra, V., Griebel, P., 1980; Reactivation of temperature-sensitive and non-temperature-sensitive infectious bovine rhinotracheitis vaccine virus with dexamethasone. Infect Immun 29, 483-488.

Pastoret, P.P., 1999; Veterinary vaccinology. Comptes rendus de l'academie des sciences, Serie III - Sciences de la vie - life sciences 322, 967-972.

Pensaert, M.B., De Smet, K., De Waele, K., 1990; Extent and duration of virulent virus excretion upon challenge of pigs vaccinated with different glycoprotein-deleted Aujeszky's disease vaccines. Vet Microbiol 22, 107-117.

Pritchard, G.C., Banks, M., Vernon, R.E., 2003; Subclinical breakdown with infectious bovine rhinotracheitis virus infection in dairy herd of high health status. Vet Rec 153, 113-117.

Puntel, M., Fondevila, N.A., Blanco Viera, J., O'Donnell, V.K., Marcovecchio, J.F., Carrillo, B.J., Schudel, A.A., 1999; Serological survey of viral antibodies in llamas (Lama glama) in Argentina. Zbl Vet Med B 46, 157-161.

Read, D.H., Sinclair, J.A., 1988; Aujeszky's disease in a dog. Surveillance 15, 13.

Reist, M., Sievi, M., Feyer, D., Schwermer, H.-P., 2006; National Survey 2005. SFVO Magazine 2006, 40-43.

Rock, D., Lokensgard, J., Lewis, T., Kutish, G., 1992; Characterization of dexamethasone-induced reactivation of latent bovine herpesvirus 1. J Virol 66, 2484-2490.

Rock, D.L., 1993; The molecular basis of latent infections by alphaherpesviruses. Semin Virol 4, 157-165.

Roscoe, D.E., Holste, W.C., Sorhage, F.E., Campbell, C., Niezgoda, M., Buchannan, R., Diehl, D., Niu, H.S., Rupprecht, C.E., 1998; Efficacy of an oral vaccinia-rabies glycoprotein recombinant vaccine in controlling epidemic raccoon rabies in New Jersey. J Wildl Dis 34, 752-763.

Salwa, A., 2004; A natural outbreak of Aujeszky's disease in farm animals. Pol J Vet Sci 7, 261-266.

Schang, L.M., Kutish, G.F., Osorio, F.A., 1994; Correlation between precolonization of trigeminal ganglia by attenuated strains of pseudorabies virus and resistance to wild-type virus latency. J Virol 68, 8470-8476.

Schmitt, B.J., Osorio, F.A., Stroup, W.W., Gibbs, E.P., 1991; A comparison of differential diagnostic tests to detect antibodies to pseudorabies glycoproteins gX, gI, and gIII in naturally infected feral pigs. J Vet Diagn Invest 3, 344-345.

Schoenbaum, M.A., Beran, G.W., Murphy, D.P., 1990; Pseudorabies virus latency and reactivation in vaccinated swine. Am J Vet Res 51, 334-338.

Schwyzer, M., Ackermann, M., 1996; Molecular virology of ruminant herpesviruses. Vet Microbiol 53, 17-29.

Schynts, F., Lemaire, M., Ros, C., Belak, S., Thiry, E., 2001; Establishment of latency associated with glycoprotein E (gE) seroconversion after bovine herpesvirus 1 infection in calves with high levels of passive antibodies lacking gE antibodies. Vet Microbiol 82, 211-222.

Siger, L., Bowen, R.A., Karaca, K., Murray, M.J., Gordy, P.W., Loosmore, S.M., Audonnet, J.C., Nordgren, R.M., Minke, J.M., 2004; Assessment of the efficacy of a single dose of a recombinant vaccine against West Nile virus in response to natural challenge with West Nile virus-infected mosquitoes in horses. Am J Vet Res 65, 1459-1462.

Smith, G.A., Young, P.L., Reed, K.C., 1995; Emergence of a new bovine herpesvirus 1 strain in Australian feedlots. Arch Virol 140, 599-603.

Stegeman, A., 1995; Pseudorabies virus eradication by area-wide vaccination is feasible. Vet Q 17, 150-156.

Straub, O.C., 1979; Persistence of infectious bovine rhinotracheitis / infectious pustular vulvovaginitis virus in the respiratory and genital tract of cattle. Comp Immunol Microbiol Infect Dis 2, 285-294.

Straub, O.C., 1990; Infectious bovine rhinotracheitis virus, In: Dinter, Virus Infections of Ruminants. Elsevier Science Publishers B.V., Amsterdam, pp. 71-108.

Straub, O.C., 2001; Advances in BHV1 (IBR) research. Tierarztl Wochenschr 108, 419-422.

Swayne, D.E., Garcia, M., Beck, J.R., Kinney, N., Suarez, D.L., 2000; Protection against diverse highly pathogenic H5 avian influenza viruses in chickens immunized with a recombinant fowlpox vaccine containing an H5 avian influenza hemagglutinin gene insert. Vaccine 18, 1088-1095.

Tanaka, S., Mannen, K., 2003, Effect of mild stress in mice latently infected Pseudorabies virus. Exp Anim 52(5), 383-386.

Tamba, M., Calabrese, R., Finelli, E., Cordioli, P., 2002; Risk factors for Aujeszky's-disease seropositivity of swine herds of a region of northern Italy. Prev Vet Med 54, 203-212.

Thiry, E., Saliki, J., Schwers, A., Pastoret, P.P., 1985; Parturition as a stimulus of IBR virus reactivation. Vet Rec 116, 599-600.

Thiry, E., Saliki, J., Bublot, M., Pastoret, P.P., 1987; Reactivation of infectious bovine rhinotracheitis virus by transport. Comp Immunol Microbiol Infect Dis 10, 59-63.

Thrusfield, M.V., 2005; Veterinary Epidemiology, Vol 1, 3rd Edition. Blackwell Publishing, UK.

Toussaint, J.F., Rziha, H.J., Bauer, B., Letellier, C., Kerkhofs, P., 2004; Effects of hypervaccination with bovine herpesvirus type 1 gE-deleted marker vaccines on the serological response and virological status of calves challenged with wild-type virus. Vet Rec 155, 553-558.

van Drunen Littel-van den Hurk, S., Myers, D., Doig, P.A., Karvonen, B., Habermehl, M., Babiuk, L.A., Jelinski, M., Van Donkersgoed, J., Schlesinger, K., Rinehart, C., 2001; Identification of a mutant bovine herpesvirus-1 (BHV-1) in post-arrival outbreaks of IBR in feedlot calves and protection with conventional vaccination. Can J Vet Res 65, 81-88.

van Drunen Littel-van den Hurk, S., 2006; Rationales and perspectives on the success of vaccination against bovine herpesvirus-1. Vet Microbiol 113, 275-282.

van Engelenburg, F.A.C., Kaashoek, M.J., Rijsewijk, F.A.M., van den Burg, L., Moerman, A., Gielkens, A.L.J., van Oirschot, J.T., 1994; A glycoprotein E deletion mutant of bovine herpesvirus 1 is avirulent in calves. J Gen Virol 75, 2311-2318.

van Oirschot, J.T., Gielkens, A.L., 1984; In vivo and in vitro reactivation of latent pseudorabies virus in pigs born to vaccinated sows. Am J Vet Res 45, 567-571.

van Oirschot, J.T., 1988a; Aujeszky's disease: vaccines and diagnostics. Vet Rec 122, 371.

van Oirschot, J.T., 1988b; Induction of antibodies to glycoprotein I in pigs exposed to different doses of a mildly virulent strain of Aujeszky's disease virus. Vet Rec 122, 599-603.

van Oirschot, J.T., Houwers, D.J., Rziha, H.J., Moonen, P.J., 1988c; Development of an ELISA for detection of antibodies to glycoprotein I of Aujeszky's disease virus: a method for the serological differentiation between infected and vaccinated pigs. J Virol Methods 22, 191-206.

van Oirschot, J.T., Oei, H.L., 1989; Comparison of two ELISAs for detecting antibodies to glycoprotein I of Aujeszky's disease virus. Vet Rec 125, 63-64.

van Oirschot, J.T., Gielkens, A.L.J., Moormann, R.J.M., Berns, A.J.M. 1990a; Marker vaccines, virus protein-specific antibody assays and the control of Aujeszky's disease. Vet Microbiol 23, 85-101.

van Oirschot, J.T., Terpstra, C., Moormann, R.J., Berns, A.J., Gielkens, A.L., 1990b; Safety of an Aujeszky's disease vaccine based on deletion mutant strain 783 which does not express thymidine kinase and glycoprotein I. Vet Rec 127, 443-446.

van Oirschot, J.T., Moormann, R.J., Berns, A.J., Gielkens, A.L., 1991; Efficacy of a pseudorabies virus vaccine based on deletion mutant strain 783 that does not express thymidine kinase and glycoprotein I. Am J Vet Res 52, 1056-1060.

van Oirschot, J.T., Kaashoek, M.J., Rijsewijk, F.A., 1996a; Advances in the development and evaluation of bovine herpesvirus 1 vaccines. Vet Microbiol 53, 43-54.

van Oirschot, J.T., Kaashoek, M.J., Rijsewijk, F.A.M., Stegeman, J.A., 1996b; The use of marker vaccines in eradication of herpesviruses. J Biotech 44, 75-81.

van Oirschot, J.T., Kaashoek, M.J., Maris, V., M.A., Weerdmeester, K., Rijsewijk, F.A., 1997; An enzyme-linked immunosorbent assay to detect antibodies against glycoprotein gE of bovine herpesvirus 1 allows differentiation between infected and vaccinated cattle. J Virol Methods 67, 23-34.

van Oirschot, J.T., 1999; Diva vaccines that reduce virus transmission. J Biotech 73, 195-205.

van Oirschot, J.T., 2001; Present and future of veterinary viral vaccinology: A review. Vet Q 23, 100-108.

van Rooij, E.M., de Bruin, M.G., de Visser, Y.E., Middel, W.G., Boersma, W.J., Bianchi, A.T., 2004; Vaccine-induced T cell-mediated immunity plays a critical role in early protection against pseudorabies virus (suid herpes virus type 1) infection in pigs. Vet Immunol Immunopathol 99, 113-125.

van Schaik, G., Schukken, Y.H., Nielen, M., Dijkhuizen, A.A., Benedictus, G., 2001; Risk factors for introduction of BHV1 into BHV1-free Dutch dairy farms: a case-control study. Vet Q 23, 71-76.

Vannier, P., 1985; Experimental infection of fattening pigs with pseudorabies (Aujeszky's disease) virus: efficacy of attenuated live- and inactivated-virus vaccines in pigs with or without passive immunity. Am J Vet Res 46, 1498-1502.

Vilnis, A., Sussman, M.D., Thacker, B.J., Senn, M., Maes, R.K., 1998; Vaccine genotype and route of administration affect pseudorabies field virus latency load after challenge. Vet Microbiol 62, 81-96.

Visser, N., 1997; Vaccination strategies for improving the efficacy of programs to eradicate Aujeszky's disease virus. Vet Microbiol 55, 61-74.

Vonk Noordegraaf, A., Buijtels, J.A., Dijkhuizen, A.A., Franken, P., Stegeman, J.A., Verhoeff, J., 1998; An epidemiological and economic simulation model to evaluate the spread and control of infectious bovine rhinotracheitis in The Netherlands. Prev Vet Med 36, 219-238.

Vonk Noordegraaf, A., Jalvingh, A.W., de Jong, M.C., Franken, P., Dijkhuizen, A.A., 2000; Evaluating control strategies for outbreaks in BHV1-free areas using stochastic and spatial simulation. Prev Vet Med 44, 21-42.

Vose, D.J., 1997; Risk analysis in relation to the importation and exportation of animal products. Rev Sci Tech OIE 16, 17-29.

Vose, D.J., 2003; Risk Analysis: A quantitative guide, 2 Edition. John Wiley & Sons Ltd., Chinchester, England.

Weigel, R.M., Austin, C.C., Siegel, A.M., Biehl, L.G., Taft, A.C., 1992; Risk factors associated with the seroprevalence of pseudorabies virus in Illinois swine herds. Prev Vet Med 12, 113-140.

Wellemans, G., Dive, M., Strobbe, R., 1976; Isolement d'un virus IBR chez un veau après usage de cortisoniques. Annales Méd Vét 120, 127-128.

White, A.K., Ciacci-Zanella, J., Galeota, J., Ele, S., Osorio, F.A., 1996; Comparison of the abilities of serologic tests to detect pseudorabies-infected pigs during the latent phase of infection. Am J Vet Res 57, 608-611.

Wittmann, G., Ohlinger, V., Hohn, U., 1982; Replication of the Aujeszky virus in vaccinated swine following experimental infection with large and medium amounts of virus. Zbl Vet Med B 29, 24-30.

Wittmann, G., 1991; Spread and control of Aujeszky's disease (AD). Comp Immunol Microbiol Infect Dis 14, 165-173.

Wyler, R., Engels, M., Schwyzer, M., 1989; Infectious bovine thinotracheitis / vulvovaginitis (BHV-1), In: Wittmann, G., Herpesvirus diseases of cattle, horses and pigs. Kluwer Academic Publishers, Boston, pp. 1-72.

Zuckermann, F.A., 2000; Aujeszky's disease virus: opportunities and challenges. Vet Res 31, 121-131.

Index of tables and figures

Table		Page
Table I.	Important members of the family Herpesviridae	5
Table II.	Situation in the EU member states regarding AD and IBR in 2004	14
Table III.	Details on some approved AD eradication programmes in Europe in 2004	17
Table IV.	Model overview for Aujeszky's disease	38
Table V.	Definitions of parameters used in the AD model	39
Table VI.	Probability of infection of the animal: Values obtained by calculation	42
Table VII.	Probability of infection of herd: Values derived from Submodel HPrev for Spain	42
Table VIII.	Probability of seroconversion: Values derived from calculation	43
Table IX.	Test performance of gE-ELISA: Values derived from Bayes model	44
Table X.	Submodel Herd prevalence: Apparent prevalence and incidence rate	47
Table XI.	Submodel Herd prevalence: Expected values for HPrev for different herd sizes	50
Table XII.	Model overview for IBR	58
Table XIII.	Definitions for parameters used in the IBR model	59
Table XIV.	Probability of infection of the animal: Effective probability of infection	63
Table XV.	Probability of infection of the animal: Values calculated for herd type	64
Table XVI.	Relative risks of infection for different age classes	66
Table XVII.	Submodel sensitivities: Values obtained for sensitivity of dependent tests	72
Table XVIII.	Test sentinels: Expected value for sensitivity and specificity	73

Figure		Page
Figure 1.	Principles of a CSF subunit marker vaccine	11
Figure 2.	DIVA strategy for IBR	13
Figure 3.	Situation for Aujeszky's disease in Europe 2004 according to 2004/EC/320	17
Figure 4.	Situation for IBR in Europe 2004 according to 2004/EC/215	18
Figure 5.	Overview of the processes for importing live pigs into Switzerland	25
Figure 6.	Overview of the processes for importing live cattle into Switzerland	28
Figure 7.	Release assessment for AD, Part I: Selection of animal	34
Figure 8.	Release assessment for AD, Part II: Quarantine and test abroad	35
Figure 9.	Exposure assessment for AD, Part I: Separation in Switzerland	36
Figure 10.	Exposure assessment for AD, Part II: Introduction into domestic herd	37
Figure 11.	Submodel HPrev: Scenario tree for infected among negative tested herds	49
Figure 12.	Release assessment for IBR, Part I: Selection of animal	54

Figure 13.	Release assessment for IBR, Part II: Quarantine and testing abroad	55
Figure 14.	Exposure assessment for IBR, Part I: Separation in CH	56
Figure 15.	Exposure assessment for IBR, Part II; Introduction into domestic herd	57
Figure 16.	Age of 3011 cattle imported into Switzerland from 2000 - 2005	63
Figure 17.	Obtained values for the probability of introduction of AD	75
Figure 18.	Cumulative distribution of the probability of AD introduction in a vaccinated pig	76
Figure 19.	Cumulative distribution of the probability of AD introduction in a non-vaccinated pig	76
Figure 20.	Obtained values for the probability of introduction of IBR into Switzerland by one single imported cattle	77
Figure 21.	Cumulative distribution of the probability of IBR introduction in one vaccinated cattle	78
Figure 22.	Cumulative distribution of the probability of IBR introduction in one non-vaccinated cattle	78
Figure 23.	Regression sensitivity for a vaccinated pig	79
Figure 24.	Regression sensitivity for a non-vaccinated pig	80
Figure 25.	Regression sensitivity for a vaccinated cattle in a non-vaccinated group	80
Figure 26.	Regression sensitivity for a vaccinated cattle in a vaccinated group	81
Figure 27.	Regression sensitivity for non-vaccinated cattle	82

Acknowledgements

My most sincere thanks are given to:

Dr. E. Breidenbach for your guidance, professional support and corrections. Thank you for the excellent supervision, your patience and that you always had time for me and my problems throughout the two years of this project. I appreciate your commitment to this project and I am grateful for your confidence.

PD Dr. K.D.C. Stärk for the scientific support, the careful reading and correction of all manuscripts, and the helpful advices. Your input as a member of the expert group as well as your encouragement for my project were invaluable. In addition, I would like to thank you for giving me the opportunity to travel to Japan.

PD Dr. FVM M. Engels for your expertise in virology, your patience and your contribution to the expert group. Your exhaustive corrections of the manuscript and your amazing skills for detecting little mistakes were indispensable. Thank you very much for your support and all the time you have devoted to this project.

PD Dr. FVM C. Griot for your participation in the expert group, your valuable comments and inputs for the manuscripts and your support in all issues. I appreciate your motivation and enthusiasm for this project very much.

Prof. Dr. M. Ackermann for your input as an expert in virology and for accepting the thesis.

Dr. G. Markov for the thorough revision of English spelling and grammar in the manuscript. Thank you for spending so much extra time for my work.

PD Dr. M. Greiner for your exhausitve review of the Aujeszky's disease model and the helpful comments and suggestions. I am certain that your contribution improved the model a lot.

Dr. L. Knopf for the thorough review of the IBR model and the valuable suggestions. The discussions and constructive feedbacks brought the model forward and taught me a lot about statistics and modelling.

Dr. H.-P. Schwermer for your inputs and answers to all my little questions within the last two years. Thank you for the review of the IBR model and the motivating discussions that helped developing the Bayes submodel for Aujeszky's disease.

Dr. G. Regula for answering all my urgent requests on the spot and that you always found time for my little concerns. I appreciate your contribution to the development of the Bayes submodel for Aujeszky's disease.

Dr. T.C. Mettenleiter and **Dr. M. Beer** for giving me the permission to use the two pictures from your publication as Figures 1 and 2 in this thesis.

All the companies and veterinary services that responded to my request, in particular Dr. T. Müller, PD Dr. M. Beer and Dr. I. Lemke from Veterinary Service in Germany, Dr. G. Marechal and P. Mennecier from Veterinary Service in France, Dr. F. Bertani from Ministry of Health in Italy, P.C. Van der Valk from Fort Dodge Animal Health, G. Cowan from Pfizer Animal Health, Dr. K. Koch from Bayer Health Care, and Dr. H. De Smit from Intervet.

V. Racloz for all the proof-reading of English manuscripts and letters within the last two years. Thank you for being such a great friend and that you always had time for my urgent corrections.

Dr. R. Hauser and **Dr. D. Hadorn** for your inputs to the IBR model and your support in all risk assessment and modelling matters.

M. Halbeisen for the support in all administrative questions and your invaluable engagement for the whole team.

My collegues and friends of the Monitoring group, SFVO, Bern, for all your suggestions, critics and inputs. Thank you all for the great time I had at SFVO and for all your support at professional as well as personal level.

All my friends for your company and your loyality through these two years when I had hardly time for anything except commuting. I am very grateful for your friendship, your respect and your affection. Most of all I would like to thank Sarah for your patience and that you were always there for me.

My parents, K. Stricker and G. Markov, and my grandmother, G. Stricker, for your love and moral support. Thank you for your confidence, trust and encouragement. And, last but not least, for financing my studies over the last 30 years.

My cat and my horse, without you, I would not be who I am.

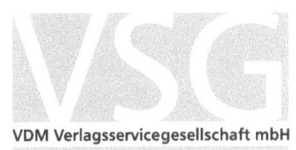

Die VDM Verlagsservicegesellschaft sucht für wissenschaftliche Verlage abgeschlossene und herausragende

Dissertationen, Habilitationen, Diplomarbeiten, Master Theses, Magisterarbeiten usw.

für die kostenlose Publikation als Fachbuch.

Sie verfügen über eine Arbeit, die hohen inhaltlichen und formalen Ansprüchen genügt, und haben Interesse an einer honorarvergüteten Publikation?

Dann senden Sie bitte erste Informationen über sich und Ihre Arbeit per Email an *info@vdm-vsg.de*.

Sie erhalten kurzfristig unser Feedback!

VDM Verlagsservicegesellschaft mbH
Dudweiler Landstr. 99　　　　　Telefon　+49 681 3720 174
D - 66123 Saarbrücken　　　　　Fax　　　+49 681 3720 1749
www.vdm-vsg.de

Die VDM Verlagsservicegesellschaft mbH vertritt

　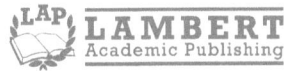　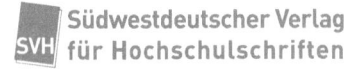

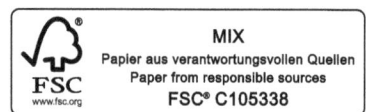

Printed by Books on Demand GmbH, Norderstedt / Germany